Averting AIDS Crises in Eastern Europe and Central Asia

Averting AIDS Crises in Eastern Europe and Central Asia

A Regional Support Strategy

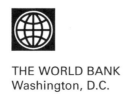

THE WORLD BANK
Washington, D.C.

© 2003 The International Bank for Reconstruction and Development /
The World Bank
1818 H Street, NW
Washington, DC 20433
Telephone 202-473-1000
Internet www.worldbank.org
E-mail feedback@worldbank.org

1 2 3 4 06 05 04 03

The findings, interpretations, and conclusions expressed herein are those of the author(s) and do not necessarily reflect the views of the Board of Executive Directors of the World Bank or the governments they represent.

The World Bank does not guarantee the accuracy of the data included in this work. The boundaries, colors, denominations, and other information shown on any map in this work do not imply any judgment on the part of the World Bank concerning the legal status of any territory or the endorsement or acceptance of such boundaries.

ISBN 0-8213-5580-5

Library of Congress Cataloging-in-Publication Data

Averting AIDS Crises in Eastern Europe and Central Asia: a regional support strategy/Olusoji Adeyi... [et al.]
    p. cm.
Includes bibliographic references and index.
ISBN 0-8213-5580-5.
    1. AIDS (Disease)—Europe, Eastern—Prevention. 2. AIDS (Disease)—Asia, Central—Prevention. I. Adeyi, Olusoji.

RA643.86E852A95 2003
362.196'9792'00947-dc22   2003057178

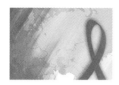

Contents

Tables

Figures

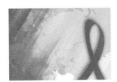

Preface

This Regional Support Strategy is in recognition of the threats that unchecked epidemics of HIV/AIDS and tuberculosis pose to many of the World Bank's client countries. It is an instrument to guide the World Bank's role in the global development agenda, which includes the Declaration of Commitment at a Special Session of the U.N. General Assembly in June 2001. That declaration reaffirmed a pledge made by world leaders to have halted and begun to reverse the spread of HIV/AIDS by 2015.

The document provides a unifying framework for the World Bank's work on HIV/AIDS in Eastern Europe and Central Asia. It identifies the potential costs of inaction, the constraints on an effective response, priority actions to resolve such constraints, and the Bank's plans for helping countries do so as part of a multi-institutional effort.

HIV/AIDS is fast becoming a threat to health and economic development in parts of Eastern Europe and Central Asia. Despite the dangers, country responses to the epidemic have been patchy and limited by widespread denial. Where actions have been taken to contain the epidemic, they have tended to be pilot efforts on a scale that is too small to make a dent in the overall course of the epidemic. Governments and civil society have started to address the problem, but they need to do much more to avert HIV/AIDS crises in the region.

The World Bank works as part of a global coalition against HIV/AIDS. It is a cosponsor of the Joint United Nations Program on HIV/AIDS (UNAIDS) and a trustee of the Global Fund to Fight AIDS, Tuberculosis and Malaria (GFATM). The Bank works in partnership with governments, nongovernmental organizations (NGOs), bilateral organizations, and multilateral agencies to support country- and regional-level responses to HIV/AIDS.

The World Bank is already active in the fight against HIV/AIDS in Eastern Europe and Central Asia. It has completed subregional studies on HIV/AIDS in Poland and the Baltic States as well as in southeastern Europe, and a subregional study is under way in Central Asia. The Georgia HIV/AIDS country study was completed in 2003. Also in 2003 the Bank cofinanced, with the UNAIDS Secretariat, a study of resource requirements for HIV/AIDS programs in the region. The Bank is also cofinancing, with the UNAIDS Secretariat, the development of a directory of technical and managerial HIV/AIDS resources, which will help countries gain better access to good technical assistance. HIV/AIDS lending operations are at various stages of preparation or implementation in Belarus, the Russian Federation, and Ukraine, and a grant from the International Development Association will support an AIDS control project in Moldova. HIV/AIDS control is included in the Poverty Reduction Support Credit in Albania. In the Russian Federation the Bank has helped develop models and estimates of the potential economic impact of the epidemic, with the aim of informing discussions among decisionmakers. Economic analyses have also been undertaken in several other countries as integral parts of lending operations.

Knowledge of the dynamics of the HIV/AIDS epidemic in Eastern Europe and Central Asia will continue to increase. That growing knowledge base will be useful in tackling the epidemic. The Bank's Regional Support Strategy will be updated as more is learned about the epidemic and how to respond to it.

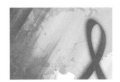

Acknowledgments

This Regional Support Strategy was prepared by a team led by Olusoji Adeyi and comprising Enis Baris, Sarbani Chakraborty, Thomas Novotny, and Ross Pavis. Lynae Darbes, Shazia Kazi, and El-daw Suleiman provided research assistance. The annexes were prepared by overlapping groups, each of which was led by a member of the study team. Gizella Diaz provided administrative assistance. The peer reviewers were Rene Bonnel (Lead Economist, Africa Region); Patricio Marquez (Lead Health Specialist, Latin America and Caribbean Region); Agnes Soucat (Senior Health Economist, *World Development Report 2004*); and Susan Stout (Lead Implementation Specialist, Global HIV/AIDS Program). The team that prepared this Regional Support Strategy consulted with and received feedback from colleagues in the World Bank Group, including Martha Ainsworth, Annette Dixon, Armin Fidler, Joana Godinho, Dominic Haazen, Keith Hansen, Robert Hecht, Chris Lovelace, Egbe Osifo-Dawodu, Toomas Palu, Merrell Tuck-Primdahl, Nicholas Van Praag, Diana Weil, and Debrework Zewdie. At various stages of preparation the team sought and received inputs from colleagues at the World Health Organization, the UNAIDS Secretariat, AIDS Foundation East-West, and the Futures Group.

This Regional Support Strategy reflects ongoing consultations among the Regional Focal Points of the eight cosponsors of UNAIDS on how to improve local capacity for developing and managing HIV/AIDS control programs, a consultation with the Europe and Central Asia NGO Working Group of the World Bank in January 2003, and follow-up communications with Keti Dgebuadze (Director of the International Information Center on Social Reforms and Executive Secretary of the Second Eastern Europe and Central Asia NGO Working Group on the World Bank).

Annex D, on nonfinancial constraints, is based in part on materials discussed at the Conference of Health Project Coordination Units held in Bucharest, Romania, in November 2002. It also reflects the authors' experiences from nonlending and lending operations in the Eastern Europe and Central Asia Region, including, but not limited to, those on HIV/AIDS and tuberculosis control.

Annex E, on financial resource requirements, is based on the findings of a work program undertaken by the UNAIDS Secretariat, the World Bank, and the Futures Group. This work included extensive consultations with country officials, including those attending a regional workshop held in Minsk in November 2002.

The preparation of this Regional Support Strategy was cofinanced by the Global HIV/AIDS Program of the World Bank and by the Europe and Central Asia Region of the World Bank.

The staff members of the Office of the Publisher contributed to the quality and readability of this Regional Support Strategy, especially Thaisa Ysonde Tiglao and Mary Fisk.

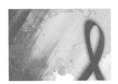

Abbreviations and Acronyms

AIDS	acquired immune deficiency syndrome
ARV	antiretroviral therapy
BCG	bacille Calmette-Guerin
CIS	Commonwealth of Independent States
DALY	disability-adjusted life year
DOTS	directly observed treatment, short-course
GFATM	Global Fund to Fight AIDS, Tuberculosis and Malaria
HAART	highly active antiretroviral therapy
HIV	human immunodeficiency virus
IDU	intravenous drug user
MDR-TB	multidrug-resistant tuberculosis
MSM	men who have sex with men
NGO	nongovernmental organization
NHA	National Health Account
NIS	Newly Independent States
OI	opportunistic infection
PMTCT	prevention of mother-to-child transmission
QALY	quality-adjusted life year
STI	sexually transmitted infection
TB	tuberculosis
TRIPS	Trade-Related Agreement on Intellectual Property Rights
UNAIDS	Joint United Nations Program on HIV/AIDS
USAID	United States Agency for International Development
VCT	voluntary counseling and testing
WHO	World Health Organization

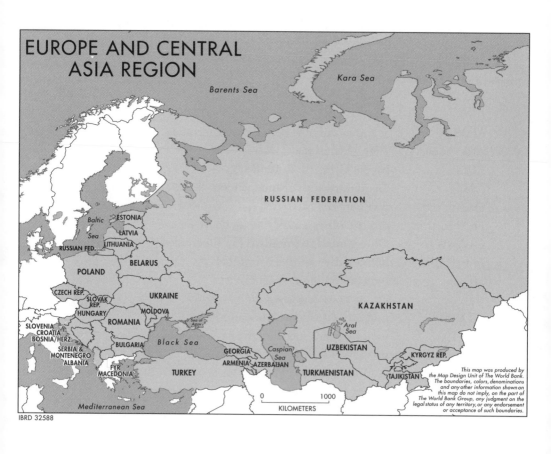

EUROPE AND CENTRAL
ASIA REGION

Barents Sea

Kara Sea

RUSSIAN FEDERATION

Baltic
Sea
ESTONIA
LATVIA
LITHUANIA
RUSSIAN FED.
BELARUS
POLAND
CZECH REP.
SLOVAK
REP.
HUNGARY
UKRAINE
MOLDOVA
SLOVENIA
CROATIA
BOSNIA/HERZ.
SERBIA &
MONTENEGRO
ALBANIA
ROMANIA
BULGARIA
FYR
MACEDONIA
Sea of
Azov
Black Sea
TURKEY
Mediterranean Sea

KAZAKHSTAN

Aral
Sea
GEORGIA
ARMENIA
AZERBAIJAN
Caspian
Sea
UZBEKISTAN
KYRGYZ REP.
TURKMENISTAN
TAJIKISTAN

0   1000
KILOMETERS

This map was produced by
the Map Design Unit of The World Bank.
The boundaries, colors, denominations
and any other information shown on
this map do not imply, on the part of
The World Bank Group, any judgment on the
legal status of any territory, or any endorsement
or acceptance of such boundaries.

IBRD 32588

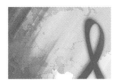

Executive Summary

Controlling HIV/AIDS and tuberculosis is a corporate priority of the World Bank Group. This Regional Support Strategy translates the Bank's corporate commitment into an agenda for action in the Eastern Europe and Central Asia Region. Its objectives are to provide a unifying framework for the Bank's work as part of international efforts to control the growing problem of HIV/AIDS and tuberculosis in the region; to clarify options for integrating effective interventions against HIV/AIDS and tuberculosis into the broader agenda of poverty reduction and economic development; to identify the main barriers limiting the effectiveness of HIV/AIDS and tuberculosis control efforts and actions to reduce them; and to define the short- to medium-term priorities for the World Bank's work in Eastern Europe and Central Asia, with emphasis on the institution's comparative advantages.

The Problem and the Context

The Eastern Europe and Central Asia Region is experiencing the world's fastest-growing HIV/AIDS epidemic (UNAIDS/WHO 2002). In 2002 there were an estimated 250,000 new infections in the region, bringing to 1.2 million the number of people living with HIV/AIDS. The vast majority of these reported infections are among young people, chiefly injecting drug users (UNAIDS 2002d). The predominant role of injecting drug users in Eastern Europe and Central Asia distinguishes this epidemic from that in most other regions.

Reported new cases of HIV are rising sharply in parts of the Newly Independent States (NIS), including the Baltic and Caucasus subregions. In contrast, the pattern is less ominous in Central Europe. Prevalence remains low in the Czech Republic, Hungary, Poland, and Slovenia.

Tuberculosis is one of the most common opportunistic infections in people with HIV/AIDS. The bacteria that cause tuberculosis take advantage of the weakening of the body's immune defenses that occurs due to HIV infection. HIV also drives the tuberculosis epidemic, particularly in highly affected areas, by promoting progression to active tuberculosis in people who recently acquired the disease and those who have latent tuberculosis infections (WHO 2002f).

Rationale for Action

An uncontrolled HIV/AIDS epidemic could have devastating consequences on health and development in Eastern Europe and Central Asia. Inaction is not an option. Fortunately, global experience shows that early and effective action can limit the spread of HIV/AIDS, as it has in Brazil and Thailand.

A generalized HIV/AIDS epidemic among economically active age groups could have the following impacts in Eastern Europe and Central Asia:

- Annual economic growth rates could decline by 0.5–1.0 percentage points.

- Health expenditures from activities related to caring for people with HIV/AIDS could increase by 1–3 percent.

- The dependency ratio could rise, putting a strain on social protection systems, especially in countries already experiencing declining total fertility rates, such as Belarus, Estonia, Moldova, and the Russian Federation.

• Household size and composition could change. The number of single-parent households and households managed by the elderly in which grandparents take care of AIDS orphans could increase. The trend could exacerbate the vulnerability of households, with negative intergenerational effects, as children are forced to drop out of school to work or take care of siblings, reinforcing the "poverty trap."

Estimation of the costs and benefits of prevention programs from selected Eastern European and Central Asian countries shows that the benefits associated with prevention programs clearly outweigh the program costs.

Adult prevalence rates for HIV vary across the region (see table 1). Estonia, the Russian Federation, and Ukraine had the highest adult prevalence rates as of the end of 2001. Countries in the region also vary in terms of income, dependence on foreign aid, and the local human capacity for tackling the epidemic. These differences suggest that while a regionwide perspective is important for identifying major issues and articulating a unifying framework for World Bank support, more detailed analyses at the country level are required to identify the most pressing local needs and the most suitable instruments for assistance at the country and subregional levels. In many middle-income countries, the World Bank's role as a financier is less significant than it is in low-income countries. Influencing policies in favor of effective interventions and using limited World Bank financing to leverage other resources can be more important than grants, credits, or loans.

Structural and Behavioral Factors Affecting the Epidemic

Structural factors increase the vulnerability of groups of people to HIV infection. Behavioral factors determine the chances that individuals will become infected. Risk is defined in this context as a probability, not a moral judgment.

Groups of people at the highest risk of transmitting or becoming infected with the virus are known as "high-risk core transmitters." In Eastern Europe and Central Asia, these are mostly injecting drug users, mobile populations, and commercial sex workers. These people in turn interact with other subgroups, known as "bridge populations"—typically the sex partners of injecting drug users and the clients of commercial sex workers. Eventually, the epidemic may spill into the general population. Everyone is thus at some risk, but certain subgroups are at much higher risk than others. There is therefore a compelling case for reducing vulnerability and supporting targeted, nonstigmatizing prevention programs on a scale that is larger than most current pilot projects. Interrupting HIV transmission among high-risk core transmitters and bridge populations is crucial if the countries of Eastern Europe and Central Asia are to avert generalized epidemics.

Structural factors that influence HIV transmission are deepseated and complex. In the medium or long term, they can be addressed through sustained, pro-poor economic growth; poverty-reduction policies and programs; control of drug trafficking; effective judicial reforms to reduce overcrowding in prisons; improvement of employment opportunities for young adults; curtailment of human trafficking; and improvement of the public health infrastructure to support testing, counseling, tuberculosis control, and other population-based approaches to HIV/AIDS and tuberculosis.

Behavioral (risk) factors are more amenable to short- and medium-term actions. These include policy support for effective interventions aimed at reducing the risk of becoming infected, improved surveillance as a basis for effective interventions against HIV/AIDS, mass communication efforts to improve awareness of HIV/AIDS among the general population, and large-scale prevention programs. Treatment programs that are carefully designed to prevent or minimize the emergence of drug-resistant forms of the tuberculosis bacteria and HIV are also needed.

Immediate Priorities for Action

The World Bank's support for HIV/AIDS control in the region revolves around two questions: what priorities to focus on and how best to approach them.

Priorities

Raising Political and Social Commitment. Efforts to control the HIV/AIDS and tuberculosis epidemics require high-level political commitment to reduce the stigma associated with HIV infection, to support possibly controversial programs for HIV prevention among injecting drug users and commercial sex workers, and to support local interventions and collaborations with civil society and the private sector. Multiple sectors and line ministries have roles to play in designing and implementing effective programs.

Generating and Using Essential Information. Much of the Bank's support in this area will be provided through analytical and advisory services undertaken in collaboration with countries and partner institutions. Cross-cutting instruments such as Country Assistance Strategies, Poverty Assessments, Development Policy Reviews, Public Expenditure Reviews, and Medium-Term Expenditure Frameworks will provide opportunities for mainstreaming policy discussions on HIV/AIDS and tuberculosis control. Emphasis would be on helping countries generate information on the status and dynamics of HIV/AIDS and apply it to their programs; identifying interventions that yield the most value in terms of preventing new infections, caring for those already infected, and mitigating the impacts of the epidemic; identifying the optimal roles of the public sector, civil society, and the private sector in controlling HIV/AIDS; and estimating resource requirements for HIV/AIDS programs and assessing the sustainability, from all sources, of such programs.

- *Estimating the Economic and Social Impacts of HIV/AIDS and Tuberculosis.* Within the Bank the Poverty Reduction and Economic Management Network (PREM) and Development Economics (DEC) Vice Presidency have roles to play in developing estimates and projections of the likely impact of HIV/AIDS on economic growth, poverty, and social inequalities in Eastern Europe and Central Asia. These estimates and projections can be used in discussions with ministries of finance, economy, and trade to enlist their support. Recent experience in the Russian Federation demonstrates that when such estimates and projections are linked to policy dialogue, they have the potential to influence thinking at high levels (Ruehl, Pokrovsky, and Vinogradov 2002) (see box D1).

- *Improving Surveillance.* Surveillance is the methodical collection of data on the level, distribution, and trends of disease occurrence and its determinants, with a view to enabling and increasing the effectiveness of the design, implementation, and evaluation of disease control programs. Both serological and behavioral surveillance are weak in most Eastern European and Central Asian countries, and HIV/AIDS programs are based on information that is neither appropriate to the highest-risk groups nor reliable as a general population estimator. Currently, they neither support program planning nor help define the dynamics of the epidemic in the region.

The Bank regards surveillance as a crucial part of HIV/AIDS control. It can support the development or improvement of such systems in every country in the region through, or in collaboration with, the World Health Organization (WHO), the UNAIDS Secretariat, and local and international research institutions and technical networks. Surveillance is so important that the Bank regards it as part of its operational imperative in Eastern Europe and Central Asia. As a result, parts of such work could be supported through analytical and advisory services to be financed from the Bank's operational budget or as part of lending operations. The Bank will finance operations in HIV/AIDS and tuberculosis control only if they include surveillance (among other technical elements), unless the client country has established a surveillance system or secured alternative sources of finance to establish or strengthen such a system.

- *Getting the Most Value for the Money.* Even with the increasing availability of international grants, credits, and loans, countries have finite organizational resources to commit to HIV/AIDS programs. Priorities need to be set to ensure that they get the maximum benefit from scarce resources allocated to HIV/AIDS programs.

Even when policymakers declare their intentions to do everything, choices must be made—the only question is whether those choices are explicit or implicit. Implicit choices are more convenient from a political perspective, since they raise no questions about tradeoffs or relative emphasis. However, fighting an HIV/AIDS epidemic, particularly a concentrated epidemic with low prevalence rates, requires effective prevention, which means averting the largest possible number of new infections within resource constraints. Evidence from the region on the effectiveness and cost-effectiveness of HIV prevention interventions is scant, making it difficult for analysts to make the case for large-scale programs financed from public budgets. To ensure that resources are used effectively and efficiently, policymakers need to ensure that negotiated priorities are informed by valid data. The World Bank will provide analytical and advisory services to help countries address these issues.

- *Estimating Resource Requirements.* Estimates of resource requirements for HIV/AIDS and tuberculosis programs have the potential to improve program planning and strengthen advocacy for better funding. These estimates need to be refined and updated periodically (see annex E). The Bank will continue to work with countries and the UNAIDS Secretariat to update these estimates and to apply them to program planning and management at the country level.

Preventing HIV and Tuberculosis Infections

Prevention of HIV is the ultimate priority for the Bank's work on HIV/AIDS in Eastern Europe and Central Asia. Based on global and local knowledge, the Bank will help countries develop and implement interventions most likely to have the greatest impact in preventing new infections. For policy and technical intervention, the Bank will work through or with partner agencies with technical expertise or appropriate institutional mandates.

The highest-priority interventions include the following:

- *Increasing blood safety.* The transfusion of contaminated blood or blood products is an efficient way of spreading HIV. Fortunately, it is possible to block this source of transmission. The Bank will help countries strengthen their blood safety programs to include screening of donors before they donate, laboratory screening of donated blood, and a move to a fully voluntary system of blood donation.

- *Promoting harm reduction.* Harm reduction refers to a group of interventions designed to reduce or eliminate the risk of HIV transmission to or from people engaging in behaviors that put them at higher risk than most others in the population. It includes the promotion of legal backing for such programs (decriminalization). Specific interventions include voluntary counseling and testing, needle exchange, and drug dependency treatment and rehabilitation. Since young people are among the most severely affected in Eastern Europe and Central Asia, harm reduction will have a relatively large effect in preventing infections among them.

- *Promoting interventions with commercial sex workers and their clients.* Commercial sex workers are among the high-risk core transmitters; their clients are among the "bridge" populations that can spread the virus to the general population. Wherever possible, the Bank will, upon request, support interventions aimed at these groups. These interventions include serological and behavioral surveillance, voluntary counseling and testing, peer education, diagnosis and treatment of sexually transmitted infections, and the promotion of consistent condom use by commercial sex workers and their clients.

- *Promoting interventions with prison inmates and ex-inmates.* The Bank will encourage the development of programs that sustain treatment of tuberculosis among inmates and ex-inmates. In some cases, such programs may require social services (as many inmates lose their rights to social program support), as well as close cooperation between ministries of justice and ministries of health. Such cooperation is challenging, but without a special approach to prison populations, the HIV and tuberculosis problem in prisons may continue to worsen.

Ensuring Sustainable Care of Good Quality

Medical treatment and psychosocial support are essential parts of care and support for people with HIV/AIDS. The range of services includes treatment and follow-up of sexually transmitted infections and opportunistic infections, palliative care to relieve pain and discomfort, and highly active antiretroviral therapy (HAART). Access to low-priced antiretrovirals has dominated the international debate on HAART. But good-quality and long-term sustained care is more complex than simply ensuring access to low-priced antiretroviral medications. Effective treatment requires that scientifically sound protocols and drug combinations be used and that patients comply with prescribed regimens. It also requires that doctors and nurses be trained and have the skills to monitor patients for adverse reactions and change their drug regimen as appropriate. Effective use of HAART requires laboratories that are well equipped to monitor changes in the patient's immune system and detect the emergence of drug-resistant forms of HIV. There is a strong public health rationale for minimizing the emergence of drug-resistant HIV. The World Bank will finance the procurement of antiretroviral drugs in Eastern Europe and Central Asia only if treatment protocols are subject to international peer review and there is prior or concurrent development of health systems to ensure their appropriate use, including the laboratory capacity and skills to support HAART. There is an urgent need for estimates and projections of incremental resource requirements for HAART in local settings and attention to the sustainability of such programs.

Controlling a Dual Tuberculosis–HIV Epidemic

The World Bank's approach to this problem will be based on WHO technical guidelines. The recommended approach for dealing with dual epidemics of HIV and tuberculosis is to improve surveillance, ensure accurate diagnosis, support effective treatment of all people with tuberculosis, and develop local capacities to design and manage these programs. A dual epidemic requires more extensive resources, careful consideration of priorities, sustained economic development, and continued support for prevention efforts (WHO 2002f).

Facilitating Large-Scale Implementation

Even as countries set up programs that are constrained by financial and nonfinancial resources in the short term, they will need to prepare for large-scale programs. The following actions are necessary if large-scale programs are to be effective:

- Developing, evaluating, and improving surveillance systems to identify high-risk core transmitter groups and bridge populations and help understand patterns of risk behaviors in order to ensure that programs focus on the major sources of infections.

- Maintaining and improving high-level political leadership for HIV/AIDS and tuberculosis control, including, but not limited to, advocacy based on destigmatization and recognition of the potential socioeconomic impacts of uncontrolled epidemics.

- Identifying legal barriers to large-scale programs and building social and political coalitions to reduce them.

- Conducting operational research, with emphasis on behavioral change among injecting drug users and commercial sex workers and their clients, to generate locally relevant knowledge for large-scale efforts.

- Conducting vaccine preparedness studies to enable countries to develop candidate vaccines suitable for the HIV subtypes prevalent in the region.

- Analyzing and disseminating information (regional public goods) on cross-border issues, including human trafficking and gender issues affecting both men and women.

- Conducting country-by-country analyses of financial and non-financial resource gaps, with a view to identifying ways to narrow them.

Approaches

The Bank's support for HIV/AIDS and tuberculosis control in Eastern Europe and Central Asia will take into account four main considerations:

- The Bank will continue to work in partnerships with governments of client countries, UNAIDS, multilateral agencies, bilateral agencies, foundations, local research institutions, NGOs, civil society groups, and the private sector to address not only program development and service delivery but also how to mitigate market failures in product development and access to commodities.

- In terms of content the Bank's work will be based on the best available knowledge from local and international sources. The Bank will work with specialized institutions to support the adaptation of lessons learned from global experiences to Eastern Europe and Central Asia as appropriate, taking into account the local context as well as similarities and differences in the stage of the epidemic.

- In terms of processes the Bank will deploy its multisectoral and multidisciplinary capacity to support priority actions at the country, subregional, and regional levels. Concerned sectors include macroeconomics, education, health, social protection, and transport, as well as institutional units, such as the World Bank Institute (for capacity building and training) and the International Finance Corporation (for engaging the private sector). Through its cross-sectoral engagement and high-level interactions with government, civil society, and international institutions, as well as through consultations with people with HIV/AIDS, the Bank has the capacity to undertake advocacy to help address gender dimensions, stigmatization, and discrimination.

- In addition to lending operations, the Bank has a variety of instruments for policy dialogue and analytical and advisory services, all of which will be deployed for more intensive work on HIV/AIDS and tuberculosis in the region. These instruments include Country Assistance Strategies, Country Economic Memoranda, Medium-Term Expenditure Frameworks, Development Policy Reviews, Poverty Assessments, and other nonlending activities such as those supporting Poverty Reduction Strategy Papers. Ideally, these instruments would include examination of the potential economic consequences of HIV/AIDS in a country, including discussion of poverty and income inequalities and their contributions to the vulnerability of societies to HIV; the main elements of the national HIV/AIDS strategy and resource requirements; medium-term goals and poverty-monitoring indicators; and short-run actions to jump-start implementation (Adeyi and others 2001).

CHAPTER 1

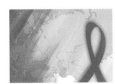

Introduction

Controlling HIV/AIDS and tuberculosis is a corporate priority for the World Bank Group. This Regional Support Strategy translates the Bank's commitment into an agenda for action in Eastern Europe and Central Asia. It seeks to:

- Provide a unifying framework for the Bank's work as part of international efforts to control the growing problem of HIV/AIDS and tuberculosis in Eastern Europe and Central Asia.

- Clarify options for integrating effective interventions against HIV/AIDS and tuberculosis into the broader agenda of poverty reduction and economic development.

- Identify the main barriers limiting the effectiveness of HIV/AIDS and tuberculosis control and identify actions to eliminate them.

- Define the short- to medium-term priorities for the World Bank's work in Eastern Europe and Central Asia, with emphasis on the Bank's comparative advantages.

The Regional Support Strategy provides a framework, not a country-by-country blueprint, which is more appropriately developed based on country-specific analyses and program planning led by the countries themselves. The Bank's approach to HIV/AIDS and tuberculosis will vary across countries and subregions, depending on the country context, the dynamics of the epidemic, the local capacity for program design and management, and the activities of local and international institutions in these areas. It will also evolve over time, as the knowledge base on what works in controlling HIV/AIDS and tuberculosis changes.

This document does not prescribe a rigid set of protocols. Instead, it emphasizes the choices to be addressed and the role of the World Bank in meeting international and national objectives. It outlines what the Bank will emphasize in support of country-led programs. It also indicates how actions may be taken, with attention to the sociopolitical context and multisectoral issues. The strategy builds on the Bank's current support for efforts to control HIV/AIDS and tuberculosis in the region.

The Regional Support Strategy has multiple audiences. Within the Bank it will be of value to the leadership of the Europe and Central Asia Region, country units, and sector units, all of which can influence the emergence of a more robust approach to HIV/AIDS and tuberculosis control in the Bank's work in Eastern Europe and Central Asia. Sector specialists and team leaders will find the Support Strategy useful in identifying needs at the subregional and country levels, in helping countries develop effective programs, and in providing high-impact support for program implementation. Outside the Bank the Support Strategy will be of interest to policymakers; regional and country officers of major multilateral and bilateral organizations that work on HIV/AIDS and tuberculosis; nongovernmental organizations; country HIV/AIDS and tuberculosis program managers; ministries of finance, education, health, social development, transport, justice, and economic development; and research institutions. These clients and partner agencies will find the Support Strategy helpful in understanding the World Bank's current thinking and future plans on HIV/AIDS and tuberculosis in the region.

Chapter 2 lays out the rationale for early action. Chapter 3 focuses on the basis for effective programs against HIV/AIDS and tuberculosis in the region. Chapter 4 focuses on immediate priorities, while chapter 5 addresses the question of how to go from small-scale demonstration projects to countrywide programs. Chapter 6 presents the report's conclusions. The annexes, which provide the context and intellectual basis for the Regional Support Strategy, include reviews of the status and dynamics of the epidemic, the economic impact of HIV/AIDS, the evidence base for HIV/AIDS and tuberculosis control in the region, the nonfinancial constraints on effective programs, and the resource requirements for effective programs to control HIV/AIDS and tuberculosis in the region.

CHAPTER 2

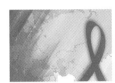

The Problem and the Context

The Eastern Europe and Central Asia Region is experiencing the world's fastest-growing HIV/AIDS epidemic (UNAIDS/WHO 2002). In 2002 there were an estimated 250,000 new infections in the region, bringing to 1.2 million the number of people with HIV/AIDS.

The HIV epidemic in the region is "low level" or "concentrated," depending on the location (box 1). In a low-level epidemic, HIV has existed for many years but has not reached significant levels in any subpopulation. In a concentrated epidemic, HIV has spread rapidly in a subpopulation but is not well established in the general population. The future course of the epidemic is determined by the frequency and nature of links between highly infected subpopulations and the general population.

In a generalized epidemic, HIV is firmly established in the general population. Although subpopulations at high risk may continue to contribute disproportionately to the spread of HIV, sexual networking in the general population is sufficient to sustain an epidemic independent of subpopulations at higher risk of infection. A numerical proxy for a generalized epidemic is an HIV prevalence of more than 1 percent in pregnant women (WHO/UNAIDS 2000).

Reported HIV incidence is rising sharply in the Newly Independent States (NIS), including the Baltic and Caucasus subregions.[1] The trend is less ominous in Central Europe, where the epidemic is being held at bay. Prevalence remains low in the Czech Republic,

Box 1. Subregional Patterns in Factors Contributing to Increased Vulnerability and Susceptibility to HIV/AIDS in Eastern Europe and Central Asia

The evidence on subregional trends in factors contributing to the risk environment for spread of HIV/AIDS in the region is weak. Secondary surveillance data that can help policymakers get a better picture of the economic and social determinants of enhanced risk to HIV/AIDS are limited. Broad subregional trends can be identified, however.

Commonwealth of Independent States (CIS) and the Baltics
The CIS countries consist of Armenia, Azerbaijan, Belarus, Georgia, Kazakhstan, the Kyrgyz Republic, the Republic of Moldova, the Russian Federation, Tajikistan, Turkmenistan, Ukraine, and Uzbekistan. The Baltic countries consist of Estonia, Latvia, and Lithuania. In these countries the number of HIV diagnoses increased from 234 in 1994 to 99,499 in 2001, largely as a result of an increase in cases diagnosed among injecting drug users. The number of HIV diagnoses among injecting drug users increased from 7 (3 percent of total) to 53,752 (54 percent of total). The number of cases linked to heterosexual contact also rose, albeit to a lesser extent, from less than 100 a year until 1994 to 4,621 a year in 2001.

The spread of HIV in the CIS and the Baltics is closely linked to the rise in injecting drug use that developed after the collapse of the Soviet Union during the 1990s. This collapse occurred in the midst of a severe socioeconomic crisis, at a time when Afghanistan became the world's largest opium producer. At the same time, trafficking routes through Central Asia were being diversified, the trafficking of heroin from Afghanistan and surrounding countries was rising, and drug consumption was increasing.

The hidden and illicit nature of drug use and the hidden nature of target populations make it hard to get an accurate picture of the problem, but the data suggest that drug abuse is rapidly on the rise. Even less information is available on the behavior of drug users, but sharing of injecting materials appears to be widespread, sexual promiscuity common, and HIV prevention rare. In addi-

Box 1. (continued)

tion, in many low-income countries in the region, shortages of disposable medical instruments, diagnostic test systems, and other means of sterilizing equipment increase the risk of contracting HIV in health care settings. The safety of blood supply is another concern.

The HIV trends in this subregion correlate well with recent economic trends, although there are some outliers (Estonia and Latvia).

Eastern and Southern Europe
The Eastern and Southern European subregion consists of Albania; Bosnia and Herzegovina; Bulgaria; Croatia; Czech Republic; Hungary; Macedonia, FYR; Poland; Romania; Slovakia; Slovenia; and Serbia and Montenegro. In these countries, a cumulative total of 16,508 diagnoses was reported by the end of 2001. Of these, 31 percent were in Romania and 44 percent were in Poland. In the late 1980s to early 1990s, Romania experienced a major HIV epidemic in its hospitals, in which thousands of institutionalized children were injected with HIV through transfusion of blood and injection with improperly sterilized equipment. In Poland the epidemic began in the late 1980s among injecting drug users, who represent the majority of all cases reported there. The number of cases attributed to heterosexual transmission in Poland has remained low and stable. In all other countries within this subregion, annual rates of new HIV diagnoses and of AIDS have remained below 10 per million people, and the main at-risk groups are homosexual and bisexual men.

In both subregions the booming sex industry, the high frequency of other sexually transmitted diseases, and drug use among sex workers suggest that sex work may play a very important role in the future spread of HIV/AIDS. Research is required to identify more clearly the variations within and across subregions in the type and determinants of vulnerability and susceptibility.

Source: Hamers and Downs 2003.

Hungary, Poland, and Slovenia. But throughout the region young people are particularly hard-hit by the epidemic.

Adult prevalence rates of HIV vary across countries (table 1). Poland, Romania, the Russian Federation, and Ukraine have the highest burdens in terms of numbers of cumulative cases of HIV, but Estonia, the Russian Federation, and Ukraine had the highest adult prevalence rates as of the end of 2001. Large cross-country variations are apparent in terms of income, dependence on foreign aid, and the local capacity for tackling the epidemic, for which the Human Development Index is used as a proxy.

Why Act Now?

Countries faced with the potentially rapid spread of HIV/AIDS have two options: delay interventions while prevalence rates are still low and intervene only once the epidemic has become visible, or implement comprehensive prevention and treatment programs early on while prevalence rates are still low (Bonnel 2000) (see annex B). Under the first scenario, development efforts supported by the World Bank could be jeopardized as a result of the economic, social, and health burdens created by unchecked HIV/AIDS and tuberculosis. Under the second scenario, HIV/AIDS–related crises could be averted through early and effective action, as they have been in Brazil and Thailand.

Denial of the problem at all levels of government has long been a significant constraint in Eastern Europe and Central Asia. Tuberculosis and HIV/AIDS were seen as affecting other parts of the world, and there was little empirical evidence to indicate that they would become problems in Eastern Europe and Central Asia. In a region going through the upheaval of transition from a command to a market economy, allocating resources to avert a "potential" problem was a difficult proposition. The situation was compounded by the fact that in the early stages, the epidemic was concentrated among marginalized groups, with little or no political clout. The rise of HIV/AIDS thus caught most of the region unprepared to

Table 1. AIDS, Income, and Development in Eastern Europe and Central Asia

COUNTRY	HIV/AIDS PREVALENCE RATE AMONG ADULTS 15–49 (2001)	TOTAL POPULATION (MILLIONS) (2001)	GROSS NATIONAL INCOME PER CAPITA (DOLLARS) (2001)	AID DEPENDENCY RATIO (AID AS PERCENTAGE OF GROSS NATIONAL INCOME) (2001)	HUMAN DEVELOPMENT INDEX (2002)
Low-income					
Armenia	0.2	4	570	9.7	0.754
Azerbaijan	<0.1	8	650	4.3	0.741
Georgia	<0.1	5	590	9.2	0.748
Kyrgyz Republic	<0.1	5	280	12.9	0.712
Moldova	0.2	4	400	7.5	0.701
Tajikistan	<0.1	6	180	15.5	0.667
Ukraine	1	49	720	1.4	0.748
Uzbekistan	<0.1	25	550	1.4	0.727
Lower middle-income					
Albania	—	3	1,340	6.3	0.733
Belarus	0.3	10	1,290	0.3	0.788
Bosnia and Herzegovina	<0.1a	4	1,240	12.8	
Bulgaria	<0.1a	8	1,650	2.6	0.779
Kazakhstan	0.1	15	1,350	0.7	0.750
Latvia	0.4	2	3,230	1.4	0.800
Lithuania	0.1	3	3,350	1.1	0.808
Macedonia, FYR	<0.1	2	1,690	7.3	0.772
Romania	<0.1	22	1,720	1.7	0.775
Russian Federation	0.9	145	1,750	0.4	0.781
Serbia and Montenegro	0.2	11	930	12.1	—
Turkmenistan	<0.1	5	950	1.2	0.741
Upper middle-income					
Croatia	<0.1	4	4,550	0.6	0.809
Czech Republic	<0.1	10	5,310	0.6	0.849
Estonia	1	1	3,870	1.3	0.826
Hungary	0.1	10	4,830	0.8	0.835
Poland	0.1a	39	4,230	0.6	0.833
Slovak Republic	<0.1	5	3,760	0.8	0.835
Turkey	<0.1a	66	2,530	0.1	0.742
High-income					
Slovenia	0.02	2	9,780	0.7	0.879

— Not available.
a. No country-specific models provided.
Source: HIV/AIDS prevalence data are from UNAIDS (2002d). Population, gross national income, and aid dependency figures are from World Bank (2003d). Human Development Indicators are from UNDP (2002).

address its impact on the health sector and even less prepared to address its impact on the society at large.

Like other regions before it, Eastern Europe and Central Asia has been slow to make the perceptual leap to begin to see HIV/AIDS and tuberculosis as more than "just" health problems. "Politicians, policymakers, community leaders and academics have all denied what was patently obvious—that the epidemic of HIV/AIDS would affect not only the health of individuals, but also the welfare and well-being of households, communities and in the end, entire societies" (Barnett and Whiteside 2002, p. 5). In many countries in the region, even the more obvious health aspects of HIV/AIDS and tuberculosis have yet to be tackled with resolve.

Increasingly, governments are acknowledging the importance of HIV/AIDS and tuberculosis and developing national programs for their control. Regional forums, such as the Commonwealth of Independent States, are making high-level commitments to fighting the epidemics. At the Southeastern Europe Conference on HIV/AIDS held in Bucharest in June 2002, governments made far-ranging commitments to preventing a widespread HIV epidemic in the subregion.

Civil society involvement is also increasing, involving not only small-scale implementation but also the formulation of country approaches to the HIV/AIDS problem and networking across countries. The Central and Eastern Europe Harm Reduction Network (www.ceehrn.lt, www.ceehrn.org), for example, provides opportunities for knowledge sharing, capacity building, and implementation support. International financing is increasing through grants, credits, and loans. The Global Fund to Fight AIDS, Tuberculosis and Malaria (GFATM) has awarded grants to 10 countries in Eastern Europe and Central Asia, for a total of $78 million in the first two years and $231 million over five years. Four World Bank–financed projects on HIV/AIDS and tuberculosis—in Belarus, Moldova, the Russian Federation, and Ukraine—are at various stages of preparation or implementation in the region. The Bank is also supporting a range of analytical and advisory services (see box 2 and annexes A, B, and E).

Box 2. The World Bank's Response to HIV/AIDS in Eastern Europe and Central Asia

The World Bank already provides support for regional, sub-regional, and country-level responses to HIV/AIDS in Eastern Europe and Central Asia. Most of the work is done in collaboration or consultation with the UNAIDS system, bilateral agencies, and, increasingly, the Global Fund to Fight AIDS, Tuberculosis and Malaria.

The Bank provides both lending and nonlending services. Its nonlending services include:

- *Advocacy.* The Bank works with other international organizations to draw political attention to the problem of HIV/AIDS. It is financing studies to inform strategic advocacy in Albania and the Kyrgyz Republic, with the expectation that the studies will serve as prototypes for other countries in the region.
- *Improving access to technical support.* The Bank is cofinancing, with the UNAIDS Secretariat, the development of a directory of technical and managerial resources for HIV/AIDS programs in Eastern Europe and Central Asia. To further improve access to technical support, the Bank works with the UNAIDS Secretariat and the cosponsors of UNAIDS to define how the U.N. agencies and the Bank can better deploy resources at the country level.[2]
- *Estimating resource requirements.* Together with the UNAIDS Secretariat and the Futures Group, the Bank is developing estimates and projections of resource requirements for HIV/AIDS programs in the region.
- *Analytical work at the country and subregional levels.* In 2003 the Bank completed studies of HIV/AIDS in Poland and the Baltics and in Southeastern Europe (case studies of Bulgaria, Croatia, and Romania); a policy note on Georgia; and a study of the economic impact of AIDS in the Russian Federation (available at www.worldbank.org.ru). It also undertook a series of analytical and descriptive tasks in Central Asia, the first of which, a compilation of country profiles, was scheduled for completion in 2003.

(Box continues on the following page.)

Box 2. (continued)

Lending operations include:

- The Ukraine Tuberculosis and AIDS Project (a $60 million loan), approved in December 2002.
- The Russian Federation Tuberculosis and AIDS Control Project (a $150 million loan), approved in April 2003.
- The Moldova AIDS Control Project (a $5.5 million grant from the International Development Association), approved in June 2003.
- The Belarus Tuberculosis and AIDS Control Project, which is at an advanced stage of preparation.

  In addition, HIV/AIDS control is included in the Poverty Reduction Support Credit in Albania.

Many other international organizations, including bilateral organizations, multilateral agencies (including the eight cosponsors of UNAIDS), and NGOs, are supporting analytical and programmatic work on HIV/AIDS and tuberculosis in the region. The discussions leading up to these projects are themselves vital in generating and building commitment among populations.

Despite these initiatives, efforts to date have fallen short of what is needed to tackle the epidemics effectively. Surveillance—the methodical collection of data on disease occurrence and its determinants, a basis for effective programs—is weak in most countries. Prevention programs for high-risk groups are also weak or too small. Political commitment is variable, stigmatization remains a common problem, and interventions such as harm reduction face legal restrictions in many countries (Burrows 2001; Hamers and Downs 2003). A recent study from the Russian Federation suggests that local policing strategies may be an important determinant of HIV risk among injecting drug users. Fear of police detainment or arrest among injecting drug users reportedly made users reluctant to carry needles and syringes, a practice associated with needle and syringe sharing (Rhodes and others 2003). Important nonfinancial factors also constrain local capacities to develop and implement HIV/AIDS programs (see annex D). Resource requirements significantly exceed existing funding (see annex E), and programs are still on a small scale. Countries need to develop and scale up their systems of surveillance and their capacities for program planning, implementation, and evaluation.

Potential Impacts of HIV/AIDS on Economic Growth and Development

A generalized epidemic of HIV/AIDS among economically active age groups in Eastern Europe and Central Asia could cause the following effects:

- An annual decline in economic growth of 0.5–1.0 percent.

- An increase of 1–3 percent in health expenditures for caring for people living with HIV/AIDS.

- A potential increase in the dependency ratio (the ratio of non-economically active to economically active people), which would strain social protection systems, especially in countries already experiencing declining total fertility rates, such as Belarus, Estonia, Moldova, and the Russian Federation.

- Potential changes in household size and composition, such as an increase in single-parent households and households in which grandparents are taking care of AIDS orphans. These changes could exacerbate the vulnerability of households, with negative intergenerational effects, as children are forced to drop out of school to work or to take care of siblings, reinforcing the "poverty trap."

Estimates of the costs and benefits of prevention programs from a selected number of Eastern European and Central Asian countries reveal that the benefits associated with prevention programs outweigh the program costs (see box B1).

Box 3. The Impact of HIV/AIDS on the Russian Economy

In the absence of effective prevention policies, the number of people in the Russian Federation infected with HIV is expected to increase markedly by 2020 (Ruehl, Pokrovsky, and Vinogradov 2002). Even in the optimistic case (prevalence rate of 1 percent), mortality rates are projected to increase from 500 a month in 2005 to 21,000 a month in 2020, and the cumulative number of people infected with HIV is projected to rise from 1.2 million in 2005 to 2.3 million in 2010 and 5.4 million in 2020.

The pessimistic scenario (prevalence rates of 2–3 percent) results in dramatically higher rates. Under this scenario:

- GDP in 2010 would be as much as 4.15 percent lower than it would have been in the absence of HIV/AIDS; without intervention the loss would rise to 10.5 percent by 2020. Perhaps more significant for long-term development, the uninhibited spread of HIV/AIDS would diminish the economy's long-term growth rate, taking off half a percentage point annually by 2010 and a full percentage point annually by 2020.
- Investment would decline by more than production. Under the pessimistic scenario, investment would fall 5.5 percent in 2010 and 14.5 percent in 2020, creating a severe stumbling block for future growth.
- The effective (that is, quality-adjusted) labor supply would decrease over time, with the overall decline due more to a decline in the number of workers (total labor supply) than to the productivity losses associated with those parts of the work force infected with HIV. This effect reflects the assumption that HIV lowers productivity by a moderate 13 percent.

Using a single-sector growth model, Sharp (2002) concludes that AIDS is likely to have a significant sustained negative impact on aggregate economic growth and annual GDP, with growth falling by 0.2 percent to a little more than 0.5 percent by 2020. Declines in population reduce somewhat the per capita impact at the macroeconomic level.

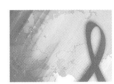

CHAPTER 3

The Basis for Effective Action against HIV/AIDS and Tuberculosis

Factors Contributing to the Spread of HIV/AIDS

Two groups of factors contribute to the spread of HIV/AIDS. Structural factors increase the vulnerability of groups of people to HIV infection; behavioral factors determine the chance that individuals become infected (figure 1). This conceptual framework serves two purposes. It helps identify factors driving the epidemic and interventions to address the epidemic at various levels and in multiple sectors. This framework is indicative rather than definitive. It needs to be updated as better information becomes available on the dynamics of the HIV/AIDS epidemic in the region.

Structural Factors

In the decade following the collapse of communism, populations became more mobile, as travel restrictions were relaxed. Social freedoms were accompanied by increased trafficking in and consumption of narcotics, resulting in the rapid increase in the number of injecting drug users. The spread of HIV/AIDS in Eastern Europe and Central Asia is closely linked with this rise in injecting drug use. The collapse of the Soviet Union contributed to a severe socioeconomic crisis at a time when Afghanistan, with a porous Russian border, became the world's largest opium producer. At the same time, trafficking routes within the region became more diversified, partic-

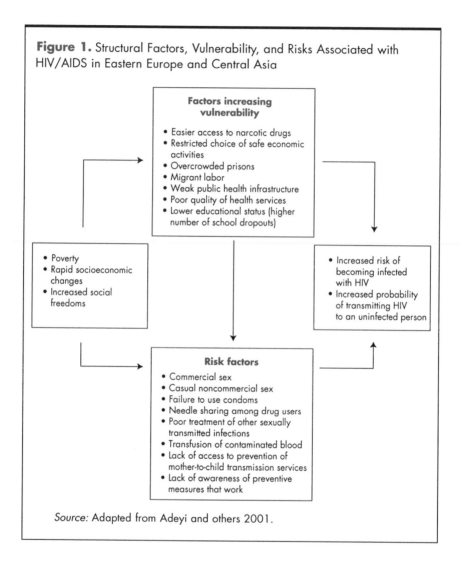

Figure 1. Structural Factors, Vulnerability, and Risks Associated with HIV/AIDS in Eastern Europe and Central Asia

Factors increasing vulnerability

- Easier access to narcotic drugs
- Restricted choice of safe economic activities
- Overcrowded prisons
- Migrant labor
- Weak public health infrastructure
- Poor quality of health services
- Lower educational status (higher number of school dropouts)

- Poverty
- Rapid socioeconomic changes
- Increased social freedoms

- Increased risk of becoming infected with HIV
- Increased probability of transmitting HIV to an uninfected person

Risk factors

- Commercial sex
- Casual noncommercial sex
- Failure to use condoms
- Needle sharing among drug users
- Poor treatment of other sexually transmitted infections
- Transfusion of contaminated blood
- Lack of access to prevention of mother-to-child transmission services
- Lack of awareness of preventive measures that work

Source: Adapted from Adeyi and others 2001.

ularly through Central Asia; overall trafficking of heroin from Afghanistan and surrounding countries to Europe increased; and drug consumption rose markedly (Hamers and Downs 2003).

The increase in drug use may exacerbate the HIV/AIDS epidemic because sharing of injecting equipment among drug users is common in the region. HIV/AIDS disproportionately affects younger people who, absent the disease, would remain in the labor force for a long time or continue to build human capital and expertise (Ruehl, Pokrovsky, and Vinogradov 2002).

During the economic upheavals of the 1990s, income inequality increased across population subgroups, changing the dynamics of social interactions. Prostitution and trafficking of women and girls across the region's borders increased (Einhorn 1998). Migration, mobility to seek work, and tourism increased sexual risk behavior, leading to increases in sexually transmitted diseases in much of the region (World Bank 2003c; Nicoll and Hamers 2002; Dehne and others 2000).

Overcrowded prisons serve as breeding grounds for infectious diseases, including HIV/AIDS and tuberculosis. Infected ex-inmates are released into society, which has inadequate facilities for diagnosis and treatment and poorly coordinates those services with prison health services (Powell 2000; UNAIDS/WHO 2002; Reichman 2002). Prisons often contain large numbers of people infected with HIV, frequently drug users, who engage in risky behaviors, including physical violence, unprotected homosexual intercourse, and needle sharing. Overcrowding, poor ventilation, and the high prevalence of tuberculosis increase the vulnerability of previously uninfected inmates to tuberculosis and HIV infection.

Southeastern Europe has several highly mobile populations, including construction workers, mariners, truck drivers, and peacekeeping forces. Many of these people are returning from or moving between countries in which the number of HIV cases is rising.

Commercial sex workers, many of whom are young, including minors, are another vulnerable group of concern. An increase in the sex industry has been coupled with trafficking in women from Eastern Europe and the former Soviet Union for sexual exploitation. In parts of Southeastern Europe the international community, particularly military and peacekeeping missions, is reportedly responsible for a significant part of the demand for commercial sex (UNICEF/IOM 2002). A recent study found that casual sex was common among truck drivers and commercial sex workers in Estonia, Latvia, Lithuania, and Poland (World Bank 2003c).

In many Eastern European and Central Asian countries, health systems began deteriorating even before the collapse of the Soviet

Union (World Bank 2003a). This deterioration probably contributed to the growth of the HIV epidemic, through transfusion of contaminated blood; poor diagnosis and treatment of sexually transmitted infections, which facilitate HIV transmission; and critical gaps in the knowledge of health professionals concerning diagnosis and treatment of HIV.

Behavioral Risk Factors

It is impossible to predict with precision the course of the HIV/AIDS epidemic in each country in the region. But review of current information on risk behaviors and lessons from other regions in which the epidemic has reached relatively high prevalence rates in the general population suggest that the epidemic could spread rapidly if effective prevention is not implemented on a large scale.

Central to an understanding of the dynamics of the epidemic is the recognition that behavior varies across populations and that these variations influence the spread of HIV (Over and Piot 1993; Hamers and Downs 2003). There are also differences across cultures in attributions about the origin and spread of the virus, as well as the nature of those groups most at risk of infection (Goodwin and others 2003).

Risk refers to the probability of contracting HIV; it is not a moral judgment of a behavior. People at highest risk of transmitting or becoming infected with the virus are known as "high-risk core transmitters." In Eastern Europe and Central Asia the evidence indicates that these are mostly injecting drug users, mobile populations, and commercial sex workers. These people in turn interact with other population subgroups, known as "bridge" populations— typically the sex partners of injecting drug users and the clients of commercial sex workers. Eventually, the epidemic may spill into the general population. Thus everyone is at some risk, but certain subgroups are at very high risk relative to others.

The most vulnerable people in Eastern Europe and Central Asia are young people, but their risk depends on their behavior, particularly drug injection and unprotected casual sex. In some cases, drug use reflects a modern rite of passage during adolescence.

For an epidemic to be sustained, each infected person has to infect at least one other person on average. The number of new cases generated by each infected person is known as the basic reproductive number, R_o (Anderson 1999). If the HIV epidemic is to decline, R_o must be less than one. High-risk core transmitters contribute more to R_o than do other members of society. For maximum effect in preventing HIV there is thus a compelling case for reducing their vulnerability (Hamers and Downs 2003; Kelly and Amirkhanian 2003) and targeted nonstigmatizing prevention programs on a scale that is larger than most pilot projects. Interrupting HIV transmission among high-risk core transmitters and bridge populations is crucial if the region is to avert generalized epidemics. A clearer focus on the behaviors responsible for most exposure to HIV in a country would lead to more effective prevention efforts (Pisani and others 2003).

Factors Contributing to the Spread of Tuberculosis

Tuberculosis is one of the most common opportunistic infections in AIDS. In the context of AIDS, "opportunistic" means that the bacteria that cause tuberculosis take advantage of the weakening of the body's immune defense caused by HIV. HIV also drives the tuberculosis epidemic, particularly in high-prevalence populations, promoting progression to active tuberculosis in people with recently acquired or latent tuberculosis infections (WHO 2002f).

The WHO describes as "critical" the tuberculosis situation in 16 of the 51 countries in its European region. All of these countries—Armenia, Azerbaijan, Belarus, Estonia, Georgia, Kazakhstan, the Kyrgyz Republic, Latvia, Lithuania, Moldova, Romania, the Russian Federation, Tajikistan, Turkmenistan, Ukraine, and Uzbekistan—are in Eastern Europe or Central Asia. Together these countries have a population of 313 million. All except Tajikistan experienced an increase in reported tuberculosis cases during the past two decades. In 2002 these countries had an estimated 433,000 cases of tuberculosis, or 77 percent of the total tuberculosis caseload in the WHO European Region, with Kazakhstan, Romania, the Russian Federation, Ukraine, and Uzbekistan accounting for more than half of those cases. The tuberculosis burden on the underfunded and deteriorating health systems in these countries is substantial.

Nine other countries in the region—Albania; Bosnia and Herzegovina; Bulgaria; Croatia; Hungary; Poland; Macedonia FYR: Serbia and Montenegro; and Turkey—are in the intermediate tuberculosis burden category. Only Slovakia and Slovenia have low burdens (WHO 2002g).

The tuberculosis epidemic in Eastern Europe and Central Asia is fueled by a combination of factors, including ineffective approaches to diagnosis and treatment, poor coverage of the population with effective treatment protocols, weak or deteriorating health systems, and the roles of prisons and detention centers as breeding grounds for tuberculosis and other infectious diseases. In the Russian Federation, 1.9 percent of the nearly 1 million inmates tested in 2001 were found to be infected with HIV; in 2002 the tuberculosis incidence rate was 30 times higher in prisons than in the general population (WHO 2002d; Reichman 2002). The high number of infected inmates creates a problem for tuberculosis control in the civilian sector, as a growing number of inmates with tuberculosis are released each year without adequate public health follow-up.

The serious tuberculosis problem in the region exists despite the availability of effective approaches to diagnosis and treatment promoted globally by the WHO. Borgdoff, Floyd, and Broekmans (2000) surveyed the literature to asses the impact of WHO–recommended tuberculosis control measures on tuberculosis mortality and transmission. They conclude that treatment of smear-positive tuberculosis has by far the highest impact on tuberculosis outcomes, with a cost-effectiveness of $5–$40 per disability-adjusted life year (DALY) gained. Treatment of smear-negative cases has a cost per DALY gained of up to $100 in low-income countries and up to $400 in middle-income settings, such as those in most of Eastern Europe and Central Asia.

Multidrug-resistant tuberculosis refers to strains of the tuberculosis bacteria that are resistant to isoniazid and rifampicin, the two principal first-line tuberculosis drugs. It usually results from poor initial management of tuberculosis and lack of application of appropriate therapy and follow-up to all cases. Specific causes include the use of the wrong drugs or the wrong doses of first-line drugs to treat tuberculosis, discontinuation of treatment before the bacillus that causes tuberculosis has been killed off, and breakdowns in the drug supply chain, which makes it difficult for health care workers to provide effective treatment regimens. Multidrug-resistant tuberculosis is a problem because there are insufficient alternative therapies available; when such therapies are available their cost is prohibitive for most low- and middle-income countries. Moreover, the spread of multidrug-resistant tuberculosis can become global, threatening populations outside Eastern Europe and Central Asia, where co-infections with HIV are even more common.

DOTS-Plus is the method used to treat multidrug-resistant tuberculosis. It is built on the five elements of the DOTS strategy, plus the use of so-called second-line drugs.[3] It is not advisable to use DOTS-Plus in an area without an effective DOTS–based tuberculosis control program in place, since doing so in the absence of technical safeguards could increase the risk of patients developing resistance to second-line drugs, which would lead to super drug-resistant forms of the tuberculosis bacteria and a major public health problem. DOTS-Plus could also reduce overall program effectiveness if it results in weaker DOTS programs (Sterling, Lehmann, and Frieden 2003).

HIV has been linked to multidrug resistance in small-scale outbreaks, such as those originating in hospitals. But cross-country comparisons provide no evidence that multidrug resistance is associated with HIV (Espinal and others 2001). Multidrug resistance appears to be uncommon in Sub-Saharan African, the current epicenter of the HIV/AIDS pandemic (Espinal and others 2000; WHO 2000a).

Implications for Policies and Programs

Structural factors are deep-seated and complex problems. They can be resolved in the medium term or long term, through sustained, pro-poor economic growth and poverty-reduction policies and programs; control of drug trafficking; effective judicial reforms to reduce overcrowding in prisons; improvement of employment opportunities for young adults; curtailment of trafficking in humans; and improvement of the public health infrastructure to support testing, counseling, tuberculosis control, and other population-based approaches to HIV/AIDS and tuberculosis.

Risk factors are more amenable to short- and medium-term actions. These include policy support for effective interventions aimed at reducing the risk of becoming infected, improved surveillance as a basis for effective interventions against HIV/AIDS, mass communication efforts to improve awareness of HIV/AIDS among the general population, and large-scale implementation of non-stigmatizing programs to prevent infections among high-risk core transmitters and bridge populations. There is a need for programs that prevent or minimize the emergence of drug-resistant forms of the tuberculosis bacteria and HIV.

Efforts have begun at changing political and social attitudes to the epidemics. They include subnational pilot projects and the development of programs at the country level. Regional efforts include the Urgent Response of Member States of the Commonwealth of Independent States to HIV/AIDS Epidemics, approved by the Council of the Health of Governments of the CIS in May 2002. Efforts have fallen short of what is needed to tackle the epidemics effectively at the operational level, however. There is a compelling case for greater political commitment at the country level. Better and more reliable information is needed to guide program development, management, and evaluation. Nonstigmatizing programs are required to prevent infections among high-risk core transmitters and bridge populations on a scale beyond pilot projects. Institutions must be developed and local capacities increased to better undertake large-scale efforts to control both HIV/AIDS and tuberculosis. Actions based on the regional context, the status of the epidemic, global experiences, and evidence-based tools currently available to control HIV/AIDS and tuberculosis need to be implemented or strengthened.

Lessons can be learned from other regions with high HIV/AIDS prevalence rates. But the epidemic in Eastern Europe and Central

Asia differs in some important aspects from epidemics elsewhere. In Eastern Europe and Central Asia the epidemic is still at an early stage, and it is driven mainly by transmission among injecting drug users. In contrast, in much of the Caribbean, Latin America, and Sub-Saharan Africa, HIV/AIDS prevalence rates are much higher and transmission is mainly through heterosexual contact (World Bank 2001; UNAIDS 2002d). It is essential to strike a balance between the transfer of experiences from other regions (such as the need for political commitment, destigmatization, a multisectoral approach, a strong role for civil society, and the application of proven technical interventions) and the crucial need for locally developed approaches. Even within Eastern Europe and Central Asia, conditions vary across countries and subregions (table 1). There are thus likely to be variations in the approaches taken, with countries with high HIV/AIDS prevalence rates needing to place more emphasis on treatment and impact mitigation. In Eastern Europe and Central Asia, where more than 99 percent of the population is not yet infected, the crucial need is to ensure that uninfected people remain free of HIV while improving access to treatment for people with the virus.

In many middle-income countries, the World Bank's role as a financier is less significant than it is in low-income countries. Influencing policies in favor of effective interventions and using limited World Bank financing to leverage other resources can, therefore, be more important than grants, credits, or loans alone. The Bank is well equipped and positioned to address cross-sectoral issues at the policy level and to support the adaptation of best practices from elsewhere. It will continue to work as part of the UNAIDS system and in collaboration with local and international agencies, foundations, and GFATM. It is already collaborating with GFATM in Moldova, where an International Development Agency grant will support HIV/AIDS control and a GFATM grant will include both HIV/AIDS and tuberculosis control activities. Such coordinated approaches are expected to continue.

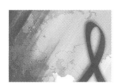

CHAPTER 4

Priorities and Approaches

World Bank support for HIV/AIDS control in the Eastern Europe and Central Asia Region is based on identifying priorities and selecting the best approaches with which to deal with those priorities. The most pressing priorities include:

- Increasing and maintaining social and political commitment to controlling HIV/AIDS.

- Generating public goods, particularly strategic information from baseline surveys (of HIV prevalence and risk behaviors) and estimates and projections of the health and economic impacts of the epidemic.

- Conducting rigorous monitoring and evaluation of prevention programs among high-risk core transmitters and bridge populations.

- Projecting resource requirements for HIV/AIDS control in the region.

- Preventing HIV infection by using the best available knowledge about what works.

- Controlling a dual epidemic of tuberculosis and HIV.

- Making affordable care and support available to people with HIV/AIDS, provided that the use of antiretrovirals is subject to international peer review and improvement of health systems to ensure quality and reduce the emergence of drug-resistant strains of HIV.

• Increasing capacity for implementing large-scale programs.

The Bank will work through partnerships with the public sector, civil society, and the private sector. It will emphasize the use of knowledge-based interventions and the Bank's capacity for analytical and advisory services at the country level. While a regionwide perspective is important for identifying major issues and articulating a unifying framework for World Bank support, more detailed analyses at the country level are required to identify the most pressing local needs and the most suitable instruments for assistance at the country level. For example, upper middle–income countries with relatively high Human Development Indexes and low aid dependency could benefit from analytical and advisory services but might be able to finance most of their response to the epidemic from domestic sources. Low-income countries with more modest local capacities and higher aid dependency ratios could benefit from analytical and advisory services and international grant assistance. Lower middle–income countries could be approached on a case-by-case basis (see annex A).

Priorities

There are five groups of priorities.

Raising Political and Social Commitment

Controlling the HIV/AIDS and tuberculosis epidemics requires high-level political commitment to reduce the stigma associated with HIV/AIDS, support possibly controversial programs for HIV prevention among injecting drug users and commercial sex workers, and support local interventions and collaborations with civil society. Various sectors and line ministries have roles to play in designing and implementing programs. Ministries of justice and internal affairs, for example, need to establish pragmatic policies on the legal status of programs such as needle exchanges and drug dependency treatment and rehabilitation, which can help prevent infections among injecting drug users. If HIV transmission is to be curbed among commercial sex workers, HIV/AIDS program workers need to have access to them, to earn their trust and operate without the threat of arrest by the police. Social marketing of condoms is needed to ensure the availability of condoms for the sexually active population, including young people. Ministries of social welfare need to be involved in efforts to support people with HIV/AIDS, ex-prisoners with tuberculosis, and mobile and socially marginalized populations.

The World Bank will support country efforts to improve local capacity, particularly leadership skills, for policy analysis and formulation of HIV/AIDS and tuberculosis control programs. The World Bank Institute is well placed to design and co-convene, with technical agencies, training programs on these issues. The External Affairs Unit is collaborating with the Global HIV/AIDS Program and the Human Development Sector Unit of the Europe and Central Asia Region on a strategic communication program that targets high-level decision-makers in Albania and the Kyrgyz Republic. These programs will be evaluated and may be adapted to other countries in the region.

Generating and Using Essential Information

To help countries generate and use essential information, the Bank will provide analytical and advisory services, undertaken in collaboration with countries and partner institutions. Cross-cutting instruments, such as Country Assistance Strategies, Poverty Assessments, Development Policy Reviews, Public Expenditure Reviews, and Medium-Term Expenditure Frameworks, will provide opportunities for mainstreaming policy discussions on HIV/AIDS and tuberculosis control. Emphasis will be on helping countries generate and apply information on the status and dynamics of HIV/AIDS to their programs; supporting interventions that yield the most value in terms of preventing new infections, caring for people already infected with HIV, and mitigating the impacts of the epidemic;

defining the optimal roles of the public sector, civil society, and private sector in HIV/AIDS control; and determining resource requirements for HIV/AIDS programs and assessing the sustainability, from all sources, of such programs.

Estimating the Economic and Social Impacts of HIV/AIDS and Tuberculosis. Within the Bank the Poverty Reduction and Economic Management Network (PREM) and Development Economics Vice Presidency (DEC) have roles to play in developing estimates and projections of the likely impact of HIV/AIDS on economic growth, poverty, and social inequalities in the region. These estimates and projections can be used in discussions with ministries of finance, economy, and trade to enlist their support in fighting HIV/AIDS. Recent experience in the Russian Federation demonstrates that when such estimates and projections are linked to the policy dialogue in the country, they can influence thinking at high levels (Ruehl, Pokrovsky, and Vinogradov 2002) (see box D1).

Improving Surveillance. Both serological and behavioral surveillance are weak in most Eastern European and Central Asian countries, and HIV/AIDS programs are based on information that is neither appropriate to the highest-risk groups nor reliable as an estimator of HIV prevalence in the general population. Some country HIV/AIDS programs and health ministries still rely on large-scale testing for HIV, including tests for certain occupational groups (such as the armed forces) and certain users of health services (such as pregnant women in prenatal clinics). Most systems are passive, relying on referrals to specialty hospitals without proactive voluntary counseling and testing. This untargeted testing is of minimal use in tracking the epidemic among high-risk groups. Current systems neither support program planning nor help define the dynamics of the epidemic in Eastern Europe and Central Asia.

Under the auspices of UNAIDS and the WHO, second-generation surveillance systems were developed to yield information that is more useful in identifying epidemic patterns and reducing the spread of HIV/AIDS. These tools are intended to be appropriate for the state of the epidemic in each setting, to change with the epidemic, to deploy resources where they generate the most useful information, to combine and compare biological and behavioral data to provide more useful information, to integrate information from other sources, and to use data to increase and improve the country's response to HIV/AIDS (WHO/UNAIDS 2000).

The Bank regards surveillance as a crucial part of HIV/AIDS control, and it can support the development or improvement of such systems in every country in the region. Indeed, the effectiveness of HIV/AIDS control efforts will be significantly reduced in the absence of good surveillance systems. Most of the Bank's support for surveillance will be provided through or in collaboration with the WHO, the UNAIDS Secretariat, and local and international research institutions and technical networks.

Surveillance is so important that the Bank regards it as part of its operational imperative in the Europe and Central Asia Region. As a result, parts of such work could be supported through analytical and advisory services, financed from the Bank's operational budget or as part of lending operations. The Bank will finance operations in HIV/AIDS and tuberculosis control only if they include surveillance (among other technical elements), unless the client country has already established a surveillance system or secured alternative sources of financing to establish or strengthen its surveillance system.

Getting the Most Value for the Money. For policymakers and analysts, an important issue is how to get the maximum benefit from scarce resources allocated to HIV/AIDS programs. Even with the increasing availability of international grants, credits, and loans, countries have finite organizational resources to commit to these programs. Priorities thus have to be set. Even where there are declarations of intention to do everything, choices must be made—the only question is whether those choices are explicit or implicit. Implicit choices are more convenient from a political perspective, since they raise no questions about tradeoffs or relative emphasis. However, fighting an HIV/AIDS epidemic, particularly a concentrated epidemic in which prevalence rates are low, requires effective prevention, which means preventing the largest number of new infections within resource constraints.

Evidence from the region on the effectiveness and cost-effectiveness of prevention interventions is scant, making it difficult to make the case for large-scale programs financed from public budgets. Even if such evidence were available, however, it would only guide, not eliminate, the need to set priorities. From the point of view of effective and efficient use of resource, it is crucial to ensure that negotiated sets of priorities are informed by valid data from surveillance that sheds light on the size and location of the problem, the cost-effectiveness of interventions (how much value for money different interventions aimed at achieving the same outcome provide), their feasibility, and social values. The Bank will provide analytical and advisory services to help countries address these issues.

Estimating Resource Requirements. Estimates of resource requirements for HIV/AIDS and tuberculosis programs have the potential to improve program planning and advocacy for better funding. Estimates need to be refined and updated periodically (see annex E). The Bank will continue to work with countries to update these estimates and apply them to program planning and management at the country level.

Preventing HIV Infections

Prevention is the Bank's ultimate priority in Eastern Europe and Central Asia. The Bank will help countries develop and implement interventions that are most likely to have the greatest impact in preventing HIV infections, based on global and local knowledge. For each type of intervention, the Bank will work through or with partner agencies with the relevant technical expertise or institutional mandates.

High-priority interventions include the following:

• *Improving blood safety.* The transfusion of contaminated blood or blood products is an efficient way of spreading HIV. Fortunately, it is possible to block this source of transmission. The Bank will help countries strengthen their blood safety programs through a variety of measures, including donor screening, laboratory screening of donated blood, and a move to a fully voluntary system of blood donation.

• *Promoting harm reduction.* Harm reduction refers to a group of interventions designed to reduce or eliminate the risk of HIV transmission to or from people engaging in behaviors that put them at higher risk than most others in the population. It includes voluntary counseling and testing, needle exchange, and drug dependency treatment and rehabilitation, as well as promotion of legal backing for such programs (decriminalization). Since young people are the most severely affected group in Eastern Europe and Central Asia, harm reduction will have a relatively large effect in preventing infections among them.

• *Interventions among commercial sex workers and their clients.* Commercial sex workers are among the high-risk core transmitters; their clients are among the bridge populations that can spread the virus to the general population. The Bank will support interventions aimed at these groups, including serological and behavioral surveillance, voluntary counseling and testing, peer education, diagnosis and treatment of sexually transmitted diseases, and the promotion of consistent condom use by commercial sex workers and their clients.

• *Interventions among inmates and ex-inmates.* The Bank will encourage the development of programs that sustain treatment of tuberculosis among released inmates. In some cases, this will require social services (as many inmates lose their rights to social program support), as well as close cooperation between ministries of justice and ministries of health. Such cooperation is challenging, but without a special approach to prison populations the HIV and tuberculosis problem in prisons may continue to worsen.

Controlling a Dual Tuberculosis–HIV Epidemic

The World Bank's approach to controlling a dual tuberculosis–HIV epidemic will be based on WHO technical guidelines. Those guidelines emphasize improving surveillance, ensuring accurate diagnosis, supporting effective treatment of all people with tuberculosis, and developing local capacities to design and manage these programs.

Dealing with a dual epidemic will require greater resources, careful consideration of priorities, sustained economic development, and continued support for prevention efforts (WHO 2002b, 2002f). Specific objectives include the following:

- Strengthen tuberculosis and HIV/AIDS surveillance (that is, conduct HIV serological surveillance among people with tuberculosis and tuberculosis surveillance among people with HIV/AIDS).

- Prevent and treat tuberculosis in people with HIV, beginning with tuberculosis testing for people infected with HIV.

- Develop models of tuberculosis prevention and treatment among people with HIV/AIDS based on field experience.

- Develop a system for referring people with HIV/AIDS for preventive or therapeutic treatment of tuberculosis.

- Provide ongoing comprehensive care for people with HIV and tuberculosis. The health sector starting point is HIV testing among people with tuberculosis. People found to be HIV–positive (through voluntary counseling and testing) need referral for ongoing comprehensive HIV/AIDS care during and after tuberculosis treatment, when many people with both HIV and tuberculosis develop other HIV–related diseases.

Ensuring Sustainable Care of Good Quality

Medical treatment and psychosocial support are essential parts of care and support for people with HIV/AIDS. The range of services includes treatment and follow-up of sexually transmitted infections, treatment of opportunistic infections, palliative care to relieve pain and discomfort, and the use of multiple combinations of antiretroviral medications, known as highly active antiretroviral therapy (HAART). Access to low-priced antiretrovirals has dominated the international debate on HAART. But providing good-quality and long-term sustained care involves more than just ensuring access to low-priced antiretroviral medications. Effective treatment requires that scientifically sound protocols and drug combinations be used and that patients comply with the prescribed regimens. It also requires that doctors and nurses be trained and have the skills to monitor patients for adverse reactions and change their drug regimens as appropriate. Laboratories must be equipped to monitor changes in the patient's immune system and detect the emergence of drug-resistant forms of HIV.

The need to prevent drug-resistant strains of HIV provides a strong public health rationale for intervention, since the emergence of such strains could make it much more difficult to control the epidemic. Key items for attention include the development of the health system infrastructure and skills necessary to monitor the clinical and public health effects of HIV therapy, including assessment of the effect of HAART on HIV–related illness and death, adherence to treatment regimens, and the development of drug resistance. Sustaining the availability of antiretroviral drugs and avoiding suboptimal antiretroviral drugs regimens are essential (Reynolds and others 2003). In addition, there is an urgent need for estimates and projections of the incremental resource requirements for HAART in local settings, as well as assessment of the sustainability of such programs. The Bank will finance the purchase of antiretroviral drugs only if there is prior or concurrent development of systems to ensure their appropriate use, including the laboratory capacity to support HAART, and treatment protocols that are subject to international peer review.

In many places psychosocial support for people with HIV/AIDS is provided primarily by NGOs. These efforts need to be better integrated into health systems. The right approach in some countries may be for a subcontracting mechanism to be developed to support NGOs with expertise in this area. In other countries government efforts through ministerial programs may be the best approach.

Approaches

The Bank's support for HIV/AIDS and tuberculosis control in Eastern Europe and Central Asia will take into account four main considerations:

- The Bank will continue to work in partnerships with governments of client countries, UNAIDS, multilateral agencies, bilateral agencies, foundations, local research institutions, NGOs, civil society groups, and the private sector to address not only program development and service delivery but also how to mitigate market failures in product development and access to commodities.

- In terms of content the Bank's work will be based on the best available knowledge from local and international sources. As appropriate, the Bank will work with specialized institutions to support the adaptation of global experiences to the region, taking into account the local context and similarities and differences in the stage of the epidemic. In the near term, interventions and approaches in Eastern Europe and Central Asia may differ from those in countries in which the main modes of transmission are different, prevalence rates of HIV/AIDS are higher, and there is a greater need for care support and impact mitigation. The main challenge is to avoid, through effective prevention, reaching high prevalence rates.

- In terms of processes the Bank will deploy its multisectoral and multidisciplinary capacity to support priority actions at the country, subregional, and regional levels. Within the Bank the concerned sectors include macroeconomics, education, health, social protection, and transport, as well as institutional units such as the World Bank Institute (for capacity building and training) and the International Finance Corporation (for engaging the private sector). Through cross-sectoral engagement and high-level interactions with government, international institutions, and civil society, including consultations with people with HIV/AIDS, the

Bank has the capacity to undertake advocacy to help address gender dimensions, stigmatization, and discrimination. Much of the work on raising social and political commitment, monitoring, and evaluation will be done in collaboration with the Bank's Global HIV/AIDS Program.

• The Bank has a variety of instruments for policy dialogue, analytical and advisory services, and lending operations, all of which will be deployed for more intensive work on HIV/AIDS and tuberculosis in the region. Instruments for nonlending operations include Country Assistance Strategies, Country Economic Memoranda, Medium-Term Expenditure Frameworks, Development Policy Reviews, Poverty Assessments, and other nonlending instruments, such as those supporting Poverty Reduction Strategy Papers. Ideally, these nonlending instruments should include examinations of the potential economic consequences of HIV/AIDS in a country, including a discussion of poverty and income inequalities and their contributions to measuring the vulnerability of societies to HIV/AIDS; the main elements of the national HIV/AIDS strategy and resource requirements; medium-term goals and poverty monitoring indicators; and short-run actions to jump-start implementation (Adeyi and others 2001).

CHAPTER 5

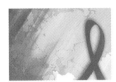

Facilitating Large-Scale Implementation

Even as countries set up programs in the short term, they will need to prepare for large-scale programs in the future. The following actions are necessary if large-scale programs are to be effective:

- Developing, evaluating, and improving surveillance systems to identify high-risk core transmitter groups and bridge populations and to help understand patterns of risk behaviors in order to ensure that programs focus on the major sources of infections.

- Maintaining and improving high-level political leadership for HIV/AIDS and tuberculosis control, including, but not limited to, advocacy based on destigmatization and recognition of the potential socioeconomic impacts of uncontrolled epidemics.

- Identifying legal barriers to large-scale programs and building social and political coalitions to reduce them.

- Conducting operational research, with emphasis on behavioral change among injecting drug users and among commercial sex workers and their clients, to generate locally relevant knowledge for large-scale efforts.

- Conducting vaccine preparedness studies to enable countries to develop candidate vaccines suitable for the HIV subtypes prevalent in the region.

- Analyzing and disseminating information (regional public goods) on cross-border issues, including human trafficking and gender issues affecting both men and women.

- Conducting country-by-country analyses of financial and non-financial resource gaps, with a view to identifying ways to narrow them.

The World Bank will support national and regional efforts in these areas, working in partnerships with governments, local and international NGOs and networks, the private sector, research institutions, multilateral agencies, bilateral agencies, foundations, and the UNAIDS system.

CHAPTER 6

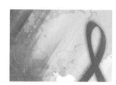

Conclusions

Countries in Eastern Europe and Central Asia face uncertain but potentially serious epidemics of HIV/AIDS and tuberculosis. Early actions are needed to avert major crises, which would negatively affect health as well as economic growth, the labor force, and the welfare of households.

There is a compelling case for greater political commitment at the country level. Better and more reliable information is needed to generate political commitment and guide program development, management, and evaluation. Nonstigmatizing programs are required to prevent infections among high-risk core transmitters and bridge populations on a scale beyond pilot projects. Institutions must be developed and local capacities increased to better undertake large-scale efforts to control both HIV/AIDS and tuberculosis.

Prevention of HIV infection and effective diagnosis and treatment of tuberculosis are the highest priorities for World Bank support in controlling these epidemics. As treatment programs are implemented, the Bank's emphasis will be on ensuring that access to antiretroviral therapy is expanded in line with effective clinical protocols and backed by effective health systems, including good laboratory services to monitor patients' clinical condition and detect drug-resistant strains of HIV and tuberculosis bacteria.

The World Bank Group will work with countries and partner institutions to ensure early action through knowledge-based programs to control the epidemics, the mobilization of multiple sectors at the country level, engagement of civil society at the national and local levels, improvement of the public health infrastructure, and support for implementation. It will mainstream HIV/AIDS control efforts through its nonlending and lending services, integrating these efforts into the core institutional objectives of poverty reduction and human development.

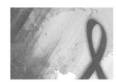

ANNEX A

The HIV/AIDS and Tuberculosis Epidemics in Eastern Europe and Central Asia

Size and Trends: How Big Is the Problem?

Eastern Europe and Central Asia is experiencing the world's fastest-growing HIV/AIDS epidemic (UNAIDS/WHO 2002). In 2002 there were an estimated 250,000 new infections, bringing to 1.2 million the number of people with HIV/AIDS in the region.

Registered HIV/AIDS cases likely underestimate the number of people with HIV/AIDS by a large margin. In addition, reported cases may not accurately reflect the possible changes in the patterns of HIV transmission in terms of the modes of transmission and the gender and age groups of people being infected. The inadequacy of current surveillance and voluntary counseling and testing services means that most HIV tests occur as part of routine screening of people who encounter the law enforcement system or use health care services.

Reported HIV incidence is rising sharply in the NIS, including the Baltic and Caucasus subregions. In contrast, the pattern is less ominous in Central Europe, where countries continue to hold the epidemic at bay. Prevalence remains low in the Czech Republic, Hungary, Poland, and Slovenia. Throughout the region young people are being hit particularly hard by the epidemic.

Subregional Patterns and Variations

The state of the HIV/AIDS epidemic in the region is "low level" or "concentrated," depending on the location. In a low-level epidemic, HIV/AIDS has existed for many years, but it has not spread to significant levels in any subpopulation. In a concentrated epidemic, HIV/AIDS has spread rapidly in a defined subpopulation, but it is not well established in the general population. The course of the epidemic is determined by the frequency and nature of links between highly infected subpopulations and the general population.

In a generalized epidemic, HIV/AIDS is firmly established in the general population. Although subpopulations at high risk may continue to contribute disproportionately to the spread of HIV, sexual networking in the general population may be sufficient to sustain an epidemic independent of subpopulations at higher risk of infection. A numerical proxy for a generalized epidemic is HIV prevalence of more than 1 percent in pregnant women (WHO/UNAIDS 2000).

Adult prevalence rates of HIV vary across countries. Poland, Romania, the Russian Federation, and Ukraine have the highest burdens in terms of numbers of cumulative cases of HIV, but Estonia, the Russian Federation, and Ukraine had the highest adult prevalence rates as of the end of 2001. Income, dependence on foreign aid, and the local human capacity for tackling the epidemic also vary widely across countries (table 1). Thus while a regionwide perspective is important for identifying major issues and articulating a unifying framework for World Bank support, more detailed analyses at the country level are required to identify the most pressing local needs and the most suitable instruments for assistance. Upper middle–income countries with relatively high human development indexes and low aid dependency, for example, could benefit from analytical and advisory services, but they might be able to finance most of their response to the epidemic from domestic sources. Low-income countries with more modest local capacities and higher aid dependency ratios could benefit from analytical and advisory services and international grant assistance. Lower middle–income countries could be approached on a case-by-case basis.

Incomplete data make it difficult to make comparisons across countries. Data on HIV prevalence in Eastern Europe and Central Asia come from two main sources. One is epidemiological surveys among specific subpopulations. Since the most affected subpopulations are often stigmatized and difficult to reach, these data tend to be incomplete and limited to small geographic areas. A second source is large-scale testing, including compulsory testing (of blood donors and military recruits, for example) and voluntary testing (for pregnant women, for example). These data are not representative of the general population.

Despite the limitations of the data, certain patterns are beginning to emerge in the region. Overall, the NIS are more severely affected than the countries of Central and Southeastern Europe. In 2001 the NIS, with a population of 291.5 million, had 234,729 cumulative cases of HIV/AIDS; Central and Southeastern Europe, with a population of 121.2 million, had 16,508 cumulative cases. HIV prevalence in 2001 ranged from 1.5 per million in Bosnia and Herzegovina to 139.3 per million in Ukraine, 594.4 per million in the Russian Federation, and 1,067.3 per million in Estonia, which has the highest prevalence rate in the region (Hamers and Downs 2003).

The Baltic countries are vulnerable to further spread of HIV/AIDS for several reasons. First, the prevalence of HIV/AIDS is relatively high and is rapidly increasing in neighboring countries to the east, such as Belarus and Ukraine, where public health conditions are deteriorating. Second, Estonia, Latvia, Lithuania, and Poland stand at the crossroads of the main East-West and North-South transport corridors linking the countries of the former Soviet Union and Western Europe (World Bank 2003c). Open borders and movement of people could facilitate the spread of the epidemic.

There is already evidence of a sharp increase in the prevalence of HIV in this subregion. The first registered case of HIV appeared in 1985 in Poland, in 1987 in Latvia, and in 1988 in Lithuania and Estonia, but very few new cases were diagnosed before 1995. Recent years have seen an exponential rise in new HIV cases, particularly in Estonia, Latvia, and Lithuania. In 2000, following an outbreak of HIV among injecting drug users in Estonia, the number of new cases increased by a factor of 32 over the previous year and the number of HIV/AIDS cases increased by a factor of 4. In Latvia the cumulative number of HIV/AIDS cases stood at 492 at the end of 1999 but reached 2,385 by October 2002 (World Bank 2003c). (These data must be interpreted with caution, since the number of tests carried out, the denominator, is not known.)

In the Czech Republic, Hungary, and Slovakia, a large proportion (20–40 percent) of reported HIV infections has been diagnosed in foreigners, often migrants from the former Soviet Union and, in the case of Hungary, Romania (Domok 2001).

In Southeastern Europe wide variations are apparent across countries, but they are hard to interpret due to weaknesses in information systems (UNICEF 2002a; Novotny, Haazen, and Adeyi 2003). Heterosexual contact is the main mode of transmission in Bulgaria (80 percent of cases) and Croatia (39 percent of cases). Moldova reports 10 times as many cases per capita as Macedonia, FYR. Injecting drug use is the main mode of transmission in Moldova, whereas HIV is spread primarily through heterosexual contact in Macedonia, FYR. The recent pattern of spread in Moldova appears to share characteristics that are more similar to those in Central European and Central Asian countries than it does with countries in Southeastern Europe. Romania's epidemic among children, which resulted from hospital-acquired infections, is a peculiarity that is not shared by other countries in the region.

What Drives the HIV/AIDS Epidemic in Eastern Europe and Central Asia?

Two groups of factors contribute to the spread of HIV/AIDS. Structural factors increase the vulnerability of groups of people to HIV infection, while behavioral factors determine the chances that individuals become infected. The conceptual framework depicted in figure 1 (see page 16) helps identify factors driving the epidemic in Eastern Europe and Central Asia and identify interventions to address the epidemic at various levels and in multiple sectors.

Structural Factors

Structural factors increase the vulnerability of societies to an epidemic. In the decade after the collapse of communism, populations in the region became more mobile, as travel restrictions were relaxed. Social freedoms were accompanied by increased trafficking in and consumption of narcotics, resulting in a rapid increase in the number of injecting drug users. The spread of HIV in Eastern Europe and Central Asia is closely linked with the rise in injecting drug use that occurred after the collapse of the Soviet Union. That increase occurred in the midst of a severe socioeconomic crisis, at a time when Afghanistan became the world's largest opium producer. The increase in opium production was paralleled by the diversification of trafficking routes through the region, particularly in Central Asia; an increase in overall trafficking of heroin from Afghanistan and surrounding countries to Europe; and a significant rise in drug consumption (Hamers and Downs 2003)

HIV is spreading most rapidly among young people in Eastern Europe and Central Asia. Adolescents and young adults account for most reported cases among injecting drug users (Hamers and Downs 2003). The virus disproportionately affects people who otherwise would have remained in the labor force for a long time or continue to build up human capital and expertise (Ruehl, Pokrovsky, and Vinogradov 2002).

The age at which young people start injecting drugs is falling. In St. Petersburg more than 40 percent of injecting drug users attending an HIV prevention center in 1999 were under 20, up from just 13 percent in 1997. Sharing of injecting equipment is common. In December 2001, 62 percent of HIV–positive men and 57 percent of HIV–positive women in the Russian Federation were between 20 and 30. Most of the diagnosed cases are males, who represent 78 percent of all registered cases, although the female-to-male ratio is steadily growing.

Income inequality has increased in the region, changing the dynamics of social interactions. Partly as a result, commercial sex work has become more common, as has casual premarital sex.

Overcrowded prisons serve as breeding grounds for infectious diseases, particularly HIV/AIDS and tuberculosis. Infected people are released into society, which has inadequate facilities for diagnosis and treatment. Moreover, services outside of prison are poorly coordinated with prison health services (Powell 2000; UNAIDS/WHO 2002; Reichman 2002). Prisons often contain high numbers of people with HIV, frequently drug users. Some inmates engage in high-risk behaviors, including physical violence, unprotected sexual intercourse, and needle sharing. Together with overcrowding, poor ventilation systems, and high tuberculosis prevalence, these behaviors make them highly vulnerable to HIV.

In Uzbekistan a third of all reported HIV infections are among inmates. In Ukraine 7 percent of 11,841 inmates tested in 2000 had HIV. In the Russian Federation 1.9 percent of the nearly 1 million inmates tested in 2001 had HIV; in 2002 the tuberculosis notification rate was 30 times higher in prisons than in the general population (WHO 2002d; Reichman 2002).

Southeastern Europe has a highly mobile population that includes refugees, internally displaced people, rural-to-urban migrants, returnees, commercial sex workers, victims of trafficking, international peacekeepers, and humanitarian workers. This group also includes people whose work involves traveling (construction workers, pilots, mariners, truck drivers). Many labor migrants and people returning from abroad are coming back from or moving between countries in which the prevalence of HIV is rising.

Sex workers, many of whom are young, including minors, are another vulnerable group. An increase in the sex industry has been coupled with the trafficking in women from Central and Eastern Europe and the CIS for sexual exploitation. In parts of Southeastern Europe there are reports that the international community, particularly military and peacekeeping missions, is providing a significant part of the demand for commercial sex. Few data exist on the sexual behavior of clients and sex workers in the region (UNICEF/IOM 2002).

In a recent study of casual sex among truck drivers and commercial sex workers in Estonia, Latvia, Lithuania, and Poland, 91 percent of respondents responded positively to a direct question about having sexual contacts while on the road—that is, sex with partners other than their regular partners (World Bank 2003c).

In the Russian Federation and many Central Asian republics, the wave of injecting drug use is closely correlated with socioeconomic upheavals that have sent the living standards of tens of millions of people plummeting, amid rising unemployment and poverty. Others factors accounting for the rise in drug use are the fourfold increase in world production of heroin in the past decade and the opening of new trafficking routes across Central Asia. The epidemic is growing in Kazakhstan, where 1,926 HIV infections had been reported by June 2001. More rapid spread of HIV is evident in Azerbaijan, Georgia, Kyrgyz Republic, Tajikistan, and Uzbekistan. In Tajikistan and Uzbekistan recent evidence of rising heroin use heightens concerns that a larger HIV/AIDS epidemic could be imminent. Already a steep rise in reported HIV infections has been noted in Uzbekistan, where 620 new infections were registered in the first six months of 2002—six times the number of new infections registered in the first six months of 2001 (UNAIDS/WHO 2002).

In several Eastern Europe and Central Asia countries, health systems have continued a deterioration that began even before the collapse of the Soviet Union. The extent to which this deterioration is contributing to transmission through contaminated blood (during transfusion) and poor diagnosis and treatment of other sexually transmitted infections (which facilitate HIV transmission) remains unknown.

Behavioral Risk Factors and Core Transmitters

Although it is not possible to predict with precision the course of the HIV/AIDS epidemic, there is reason to anticipate its rapid spread in the region. Concern over the spread of the epidemic is based on a review of current information on risk behaviors and the lessons of experience in regions in which the epidemic has reached relatively high prevalence rates in the general population. Central to an understanding of the dynamics of the epidemic is the recognition that behaviors vary across populations and that these variations affect the spread of HIV (Over and Piot 1993; Hamers and Downs 2003).

Risk is the probability of becoming infected. It is not a judgment about the morality of a particular behavior. People at highest risk of transmitting or becoming infected with the virus are high-risk core transmitters. In Eastern Europe and Central Asia, high-risk core transmitters are mostly injecting drug users, mobile populations, and commercial sex workers. High-risk core transmitters in turn interact with other subgroups that have a moderate risk of becoming infected or transmitting the virus. These are the so-called bridge populations, typically the sex partners of injecting drug users and the clients of commercial sex workers. Eventually, the epidemic may spill into the general population.

For an epidemic to be sustained, each infected person has to infect at least one other person on average. The number of new cases generated by each infected person is known as the basic reproductive number, R_0 (Anderson 1999). If the HIV epidemic is to decline, R_0 must be less than one. High-risk core transmitters contribute more to R_0 than do other members of the society. There is thus a compelling case to provide targeted, nondiscriminatory prevention programs (Hamers and Downs 2003) on a scale that is larger than the current pilot projects.

Injecting Drug Use

The HIV/AIDS epidemic in Eastern Europe and Central Asia is linked to the surge in injecting drug use among young people. Estimates vary, but most indicate that injecting drug users account for 70–90 percent of new HIV infections. Most of these people appear to have contracted the virus through contaminated needles.

Studies measuring HIV prevalence among injecting drug users reveal prevalence rates of more than 50 percent in Svetlogorsk (Belarus) and in Irkutsk, Kaliningrad, Togliatti City, and Tver (the Russian Federation). Prevalence rates of more than 30 percent were reported in Poltava (Ukraine) and Rostov, Samara, and St. Petersburg (the Russian Federation). Prevalence rates of more than 15 percent were found in Minsk (Belarus), Moldova, Ekaterinburg (the Russian Federation), and Kharkiv (Ukraine). HIV prevalence remains low among injecting drug users in most Central and Southeastern European countries (Rhodes, Lowndes, and others 2002).

Studies provide reason for significant concern in many of these countries. In the Russian Federation, for example, between September and October 2001, 426 injecting drug users were tested for HIV in Togliatti City, Samara Oblast. Of those tested, 56 percent had HIV antibodies; 74 percent of those with antibodies were unaware of their positive status. The high prevalence of HIV and a recent increase in HIV detected through routine tests since 2000 suggest that an explosive epidemic has occurred among injecting drug users in Togliatti City. This finding has urgent implications for maximizing the distribution of sterile injecting equipment as well as enhancing sexual risk reduction. Recognizing that similar explosive epidemics could be taking place in other Russian cities, the authors of the study recommended communitywide HIV prevention coverage supported by city and state policies oriented to harm reduction (Rhodes and others 2002).

These worrisome trends require rapid interventions. Most initiatives have focused on noninjecting or frequent injecting drug users. Infrequent injectors who have not yet developed fixed injection patterns have been largely ignored. Targeting infrequent injectors, however, may be crucial to controlling the epidemic. Follow-up studies of young injectors who only recently began injecting show a high incidence of infection within the first three years of injecting. A recent WHO rapid assessment report in St. Petersburg reveals that new and random injectors are most vulnerable to HIV. Effectively targeting this population could control the growth of the injecting drug user population (Defy 2002).

Infrequent injectors are a difficult population to target, however, because they stand between two worlds. Many do not yet fully identify themselves as injecting drug users and therefore have greater fear of and attach greater stigma to harm reduction strategies, such as needle exchange programs. Limited contact with drug networks may also limit their awareness of outreach programs. Whereas frequent injectors can easily be reached where drug prevention schemes and street-outreach exist, infrequent users form a more hidden population.

Unprotected casual sex among injecting drug users increases the rate of transmission. Little empirical evidence is available on patterns of sexual behavior and condom use among injecting drug users, but the majority of injecting drug users are believed to be sexually active.

Drug injecting and the sharing of injecting equipment remain the most important risk factors for sex workers. But the proportion of newly detected HIV cases from heterosexual transmission appears to be rising in places in which the incidence of HIV among injecting drug users is growing. In Odessa and Kaliningrad, for example, the proportion of new cases associated with sexual transmission rose from 5–10 percent in 1996 to 30–35 percent in 2001 (Rhodes, Platt, Davis, Filatova, and Sarang 2002). At the same time, the proportion of new cases among injecting drug users declined from about 90 percent in 1996 to 65 percent in 2001. The male-to-female ratio of reported cases declined from 4:1 to 2:1 between 1987 and 2001, suggesting that young women are increasingly at risk of contracting HIV through sexual contact with an injecting drug user partner, sexual contact with a client, or injecting drug use, which is growing among women.

Low awareness and unsafe behavior among injecting drug users, including the sharing of injecting equipment, are important reasons why the epidemic has spread so rapidly. In Belarus and Ukraine, where the epidemic appeared earliest, an increasing share of new infections is now occurring through sexual—overwhelmingly heterosexual—transmission.

Data based on the October 2001 Russia Longitudinal Monitoring Survey indicate a strong potential for rapid heterosexual spread of HIV in the Russian Federation (Vannappagari and Ryder 2002):

- One third of all 14- to 20-year-old respondents reported being sexually active during the previous year, with the proportion higher among men than women. The average age at first intercourse has declined.

- Within the 14- to 20-age group, 75 percent of sexually active respondents reported having a friend or casual acquaintance as their current partner. Among all sexually active 14- to 20-year-olds, 44 percent did not use a condom the last time they had sex.

• Among those who had sex with a casual acquaintance, 48 percent of 14- to 20-year-olds, 36.5 percent of 21- to 30-year-olds, 61.3 percent of 31- to 40-year-olds, and 69 percent of 41- to 49-year-olds did not use a condom during the most recent sexual act. Among those who had sex in exchange for money or gifts, 35.6 percent of 21- to 30-year-olds and 43.5 percent of 41- to 49-year-olds did not use a condom.

• The male-to-female ratio among newly detected HIV cases fell from 4:1 in the late 1990s to 2:1 in 2001, indicating that girls and young women are increasingly at risk of HIV infection. The rise in prostitution and the common practice of unprotected casual sex are contributing to the spread of HIV beyond the drug-user subpopulation.

Sexually Transmitted Infections

Another important risk factor is the high prevalence of sexually transmitted infections in many parts of Eastern Europe and Central Asia. Certain sexually transmitted infections increase the probability of HIV transmission during unprotected sex. The rates of sexually transmitted diseases in the Russian Federation have remained at epidemic levels for the past decade. In 1999, 188 cases of syphilis and 176 cases of gonorrhea per 100,000 people were reported—128 and 24 times higher than the corresponding figures in Western European countries—and rates are even higher in many regions of the Russian Federation. The incidence of sexually transmitted infections among adolescents is continuing to rise in parts of the country.

Commercial Sex

Commercial sex is on the rise in the region, with an east-to-west migration of sex workers (Dehne and others 2000). In Plovidv, Bulgaria, 13 percent of 200 prostitutes surveyed were Russian and a quarter were on their way to Western Europe or Turkey (Tchoudomirova, Domeika, and Mardh 1997).

A high prevalence of sexually transmitted diseases in the general population and specifically among sex workers indicates a high potential for transmission of HIV through sexual contact between commercial sex workers and their partners. In the Russian Federation, among 70 street prostitutes participating in a voluntary anonymous study in Moscow, 44 percent were injecting drug users, 31 percent had syphilis, and 20 percent never used condoms. Overall 30–60 percent of Russian sex workers are estimated to inject drugs. Estimates are slightly lower in Southeastern Europe, where 22 percent of sex workers in Serbia and 30 percent in Albania are estimated to inject drugs. Among female injecting drug users, 20–50 percent in Eastern Europe and 10–25 percent in Central Asia are estimated to work as sex workers (Rhodes, Platt, and others 2002). The booming sex industry, the high frequency of other sexually transmitted diseases, and the high rate of drug use among prostitutes suggest that prostitution may play an important role in the future spread of HIV/AIDS in Eastern Europe and Central Asia.

Tuberculosis and HIV/AIDS

Tuberculosis is caused by *Mycobacterium tuberculosis*, which is transmitted through droplets released into the air by infected people. About a third of the world's population has latent tuberculosis, from which there is lifelong risk of reactivation.

About 95 percent of people infected with tuberculosis initially enter a latent phase, during which the infection goes unnoticed. In about 5 percent of cases, the initial infection progresses directly to pulmonary tuberculosis; organs other than the lungs can also be involved (extrapulmonary tuberculosis). Serious outcomes of the initial infection are more frequent in infants, adolescents, and young adults. In the absence of effective treatment for active disease, a chronic wasting course is usual and death ultimately occurs (Daniel 1991).

Jack (2001) argues for public intervention on efficiency grounds, by identifying public goods attributes of tuberculosis control, externalities in its consumption, and supply-side failures. Tuberculosis control also serves the important cause of reducing poverty.

Tuberculosis with HIV co-infection is a major emerging health problem in developing countries. People with HIV/AIDS are particularly susceptible to opportunistic infections, namely, tuberculosis, pneumonia, and diarrhea.

Tuberculosis is easily diagnosed and is usually treatable with antibiotics, at a cost of about $10–$20 a patient. Yet it remains a major cause of sickness and death in people with HIV/AIDS, among whom the lifetime risk of developing the disease is 5–10 times that of people without HIV/AIDS. HIV is the most powerful known risk factor for reactivation of latent tuberculosis infection to active disease; people with HIV who become infected with *Mycobacterium tuberculosis* rapidly progress to active tuberculosis. Tuberculosis-HIV co-infection also undermines treatment and care, reduces survival substantially, and increases healthcare costs. The burden will be higher in countries that do not meet WHO targets of at least 70 percent detection of new smear-positive cases and an 85 percent cure rate with DOTS coverage, a category into which the Russian Federation and most CIS countries fall (WHO 2002b, d, f, g).

At the regional level the WHO describes as "critical" the tuberculosis situation in 16 of the 51 countries in its European region, all of which are in Eastern Europe and Central Asia: Armenia, Azerbaijan, Belarus, Estonia, Georgia, Kazakhstan, the Kyrgyz Republic, Latvia, Lithuania, Moldova, Romania, the Russian Federation, Tajikistan, Turkmenistan, Ukraine, and Uzbekistan. Together these countries, with a combined population of 313 million, had an estimated 433,000 cases of tuberculosis in 2002, or 77 percent of the total tuberculosis caseload in the European Region of the WHO. The estimated number of tuberculosis cases in these countries has risen during the past 10–20 years. Notification has also risen (except in Tajikistan), and the tuberculosis burden has grown. Five countries—Kazakhstan, Romania, the Russian Federation, Ukraine, and Uzbekistan—account for more than half of the tuberculosis burden in the European Region of the WHO.

Eight other Eastern Europe and Central Asia countries—Albania; Bosnia and Herzegovina; Bulgaria; Croatia; Hungary; Poland; Macedonia, FYR; Serbia and Montenegro; and Turkey—are in the intermediate tuberculosis burden category. In the region only Slovakia and Slovenia have a low tuberculosis burden (WHO 2002g).

The tuberculosis problem is being fueled by a combination of factors, including poverty (Vinokur and others 2001), ineffective approaches to diagnosis and treatment, poor coverage of the population with effective treatment protocols, weak or deteriorating health systems, and the roles of prisons as breeding grounds for infectious diseases (figure A1). In the Russian Federation case rates and death rates among inmates are 10 times higher than in the civilian sector. The case notification rate in the penitentiary system in 2000 was 3,118 per 100,000 convicts and people under criminal investigation. This high rate of tuberculosis among the prison population represents a problem for tuberculosis control in the civilian sector, as a growing number of inmates with tuberculosis are being released from prison. The prison system serves as one of the epidemiological pumps for the tuberculosis epidemic, helping breed a pool of infected people who are then released into the general population with no guarantee of follow-up or adequate treatment by health facilities that serve the population at large.

Despite the availability of cost-effective approaches to diagnosis and treatment, tuberculosis remains a serious problem in Eastern Europe and Central Asia. Borgdoff, Floyd, and Broekmans (2000) reviewed the literature on the impact of tuberculosis control measures on mortality and transmission and constraints to scaling up. They concluded that treatment of smear-positive tuberculosis using DOTS has by far the greatest impact, with a cost-effectiveness of $5–$40 per DALY gained. Treatment of smear-negative cases has a cost per DALY gained of up to $100 in low-income countries and up to $400 in middle-income settings.

Multidrug-Resistant Tuberculosis

Multidrug-resistant tuberculosis is caused by strains of the tuberculosis bacteria that are resistant to at least isoniazid and rifampicin,

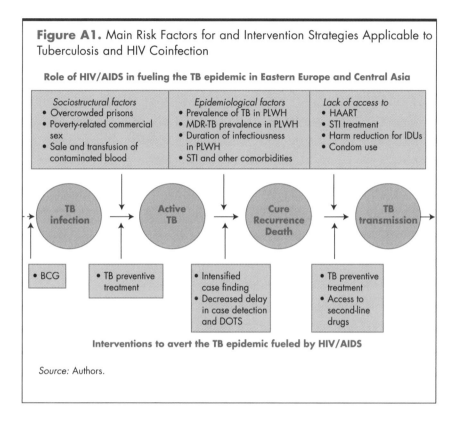

Figure A1. Main Risk Factors for and Intervention Strategies Applicable to Tuberculosis and HIV Coinfection

Role of HIV/AIDS in fueling the TB epidemic in Eastern Europe and Central Asia

Sociostructural factors
- Overcrowded prisons
- Poverty-related commercial sex
- Sale and transfusion of contaminated blood

Epidemiological factors
- Prevalence of TB in PLWH
- MDR-TB prevalence in PLWH
- Duration of infectiousness in PLWH
- STI and other comorbidities

Lack of access to
- HAART
- STI treatment
- Harm reduction for IDUs
- Condom use

TB infection → Active TB → Cure Recurrence Death → TB transmission

- BCG
- TB preventive treatment
- Intensified case finding
- Decreased delay in case detection and DOTS
- TB preventive treatment
- Access to second-line drugs

Interventions to avert the TB epidemic fueled by HIV/AIDS

Source: Authors.

the two principal first-line drugs used in combination chemotherapy. It results from poor management of drug-sensitive tuberculosis, a big problem that arises from failure to manage a smaller problem effectively. It is the result of one or more failures in the disease control or broader health care system, including the use of incorrect drugs or incorrect doses of the right drugs to treat tuberculosis; discontinuation of treatment before the bacteria that cause tuberculosis have been killed off, making it possible for them to develop into stronger versions of the same bacteria; and breakdowns in the drug supply chain, which make it difficult for doctors, nurses, and other health care workers to provide the right treatment.

Cross-country comparisons indicate that the multidrug-resistant rate among previously untreated cases is inversely correlated with treatment success under short-course chemotherapy (Dye and others 2002). The straightforward conclusion is that high cure rates have prevented the emergence of resistance in countries that have effectively used short-course chemotherapy. Cure rates of more than 90 percent can be achieved under such chemotherapy; if few patients fail treatment, fewer still can develop resistance. High rates of resistance tend to be associated with low treatment success. In Ivanovo Oblast, in the Russian Federation, the reported treatment success for patients carrying fully sensitive strains is 63 percent. With a cure rate this low, it is not surprising that 9 percent of new tuberculosis cases are multidrug resistant (Espinal and others 2000).

HIV–Related Tuberculosis

Tuberculosis is one of the most common opportunistic infections in people with AIDS. HIV also drives the tuberculosis epidemic, particularly in areas in which the prevalence of the virus is high. HIV promotes progression to active tuberculosis in both people with recently acquired and people with latent tuberculosis infections (WHO 2002b, f). It has been linked to multidrug resistance in small-scale outbreaks, such as those originating in hospitals, but there is no evidence that multidrug resistance is associated with HIV in cross-country comparisons. Multidrug resistance appears to be uncommon in Sub-Saharan Africa, the current epicenter of the HIV/AIDS pandemic (Espinal and others 2000 2001; WHO 2000).

The serious tuberculosis problems in Eastern Europe and Central Asia stem in part from the difficulties of the transition from the Soviet era approaches to contemporary practices. Health systems in most of the former Soviet republics experienced major destabilization and underinvestment, and the quality of care is poor, a legacy of the late Soviet era (McKee, Healy, and Falkingham 2002; Reichman 2002). The centrally planned Soviet tuberculosis control system had its successes, but the approach was costly because of overreliance on mass x-ray screening for diagnosis and on lengthy hospitalizations for treatment. Nonetheless, the system was held in high esteem by the Soviet health establishment, partly because the tuberculosis burden in the late Soviet era was not the problem it became in the 1990s, according to official Soviet data. In addition, incentives strongly favored the maintenance of large tuberculosis hospitals, as financing for tuberculosis services was based on the number of beds. An input-driven incentive system does not improve performance on the basis of outcomes. Furthermore, at least one generation of medical practitioners had much to lose from the rapid change of approach from the familiar to the new.

As a result of these factors, despite several pilot projects in the region, most countries have not come close to nationwide implementation of internationally recognized approaches to tuberculosis control. A large majority of the population still receives mostly inappropriate diagnostic and treatment services of uncertain quality, with wide variations across and within countries—a perfect scenario for breeding multidrug-resistant tuberculosis (Reichman 2002). In Uzbekistan, for example, the failing tuberculosis system is contributing to some of the highest rates of multidrug-resistant tuberculosis in the world, with 13 percent of new patients at Médecins Sans Frontières clinics in the Karakalpakstan region presenting with multidrug-resistant tuberculosis. In addition to drug resistance, the deteriorating Soviet-era system has created a large pool of patients who previously received more than a month of tuberculosis treatment (so-called retreatment cases). These cases make up about half of the smear-positive cases seen in the Médecins Sans Frontières program, less than 10 percent of whom received DOTS in the past. More than 40 percent of these retreatment cases have multidrug-resistant tuberculosis (Cox and Hargreaves 2003).

Controlling Tuberculosis in an Era of Dual Infection with HIV

For many years people involved primarily with tackling tuberculosis and those involved primarily with tackling HIV/AIDS pursued largely separate courses. Separate funding of tuberculosis and HIV/AIDS programs often maintained these separate courses (WHO 2002f). In Eastern Europe and Central Asia there is a strong tradition of vertical programs.

A new Strategic Framework to Decrease the Burden of Tuberculosis/HIV (WHO 2002) represents a unified health sector strategy to control HIV–related tuberculosis as an integral part of the strategy for fighting HIV/AIDS. Efforts to control tuberculosis among people with HIV have focused mainly on implementing the DOTS strategy for tuberculosis control—that is, identifying and curing infectious tuberculosis cases among people presenting at general health services. This strategy targets the final step in the sequence of events by which HIV fuels tuberculosis, namely, the transmission of *Mycobacterium tuberculosis* infection.

The expanded scope of the new strategy for tuberculosis control in high HIV prevalence populations includes interventions against tuberculosis (intensified case finding and cure and tuberculosis preventive treatment) and interventions against HIV (and therefore indirectly tuberculosis). These interventions include promotion of condoms, treatment of sexually transmitted diseases, promotion of safe injecting drug use, and HAART. Although the main focus of the strategy is on Sub-Saharan Africa, which bears the heaviest burden of HIV–related tuberculosis, it may be relevant to parts of Eastern Europe and Central Asia with particularly high concentrations of tuberculosis, such as prisons in the Russian Federation. The priority is to improve surveillance and ensure accurate diagnosis and effective treatment among members of risk groups. A coherent health service response to tuberculosis and HIV includes criteria for determining priority interventions; poverty alleviation; an attempt to deal with market failure; and estimates and use in program planning of the cost and cost-effectiveness of interventions (WHO 2002f).

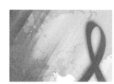

ANNEX B

The Potential Economic, Poverty, and Human Development Impacts of HIV/AIDS in Eastern Europe and Central Asia

This annex describes the potential impact of the HIV/AIDS epidemic in Eastern Europe and Central Asia on the economy, society, community, and households. Economic impact refers to the effects on macroeconomic and microeconomic indicators, such as economic growth, per capita income, the Gini coefficient,[4] labor supply and productivity, public and private consumption, and domestic savings. Social impact refers to the effects on social reproductive labor (for example, parenting); social cohesion; and the organization of communities and households.

Economic and social impact analyses are based on the premise that once the HIV/AIDS epidemic begins to spread, certain consequences are likely that are not evident in the early stages of the epidemic. Without an accelerated response to control the spread of the disease, the epidemic could move from concentration within high-risk groups to a generalized epidemic transmitted predominantly through heterosexual contact.

Over time people with HIV develop full-blown AIDS, the number of people with HIV increases, and the impacts of taking care of people with AIDS and AIDS deaths among people in the productive age groups of 15–50 is felt at various levels of the economy and society (table B1). Estimation of the potential economic and social impacts is based on pro-

Table B1. Economic and Social Impact of HIV/AIDS, by Level, Time, and Degree

LEVEL OF IMPACT	TIME OF IMPACT	DEGREE OF IMPACT	EVIDENCE OF IMPACT
Individual	Early (immediate)	Always severe; varies by age and gender.	Death and illness
Household	Early, middle (1–5 years), and late (10 years and beyond, intergenerational)	Severe emotional, variable financial depending on socioeconomic status, gender, ethnicity, and other social variable.	Household studies suggest that orphans and the elderly are especially affected.
Community	Early, middle, and late	Depends on scale and resource base of community but likely to be long term and profound, albeit not necessarily easy to see.	Services for orphans and the elderly and local service provision are affected.
Production unit/ institution	Middle and late	Depends on nature of organization's or institution's activities or type of production and labor mix.	Yes
Sector	Late	Depends on location, use of labor.	Some evidence exists, but it is limited.
Nation	Late	Economic impact is probably slight; other effects may be present.	No empirical evidence, only economic models and anecdotal evidence about effects on government infrastructure

Source: Barnett and Whiteside 2002.

jections and evidence from other regions of the world that had low HIV prevalence rates but are now facing a generalized HIV/AIDS epidemic.

Macroeconomic Impact of HIV/AIDS

Maintaining a healthy rate of economic growth is an important macroeconomic policy objective. In addition, technological innovation and development are important for countries to maintain their economic edge and comparative advantage. Human capital formation is critical for sustaining economic growth and development.

By increasing illness and death among people of productive age, HIV/AIDS has the potential to negatively affect population dynamics, labor supply, and productivity; raise public and private consumption; and reduce income and savings. With a lower savings rate, the rate of investment is likely to fall, reinforcing the decline in economic growth.

Estimating the effect of HIV/AIDS on economic growth requires using current prevalence rates and assumptions about future incidence rates to project the number of future illnesses and deaths. Once these projections are made, estimates of demographic impacts, health expenditures, labor supply and productivity, and other economic parameters can be made. These parameters are then used to model economic growth scenarios with and without HIV/AIDS.

About a dozen studies look at the impact of HIV/AIDS on economic growth (table B2). Only two are specific to the Eastern Europe and Central Asia Region, both of which focus on the Russian Federation (box B1).

Although these studies used different projection scenarios, all of them show that HIV/AIDS has the potential to reduce economic growth. The impact on GDP per capita is less clear and depends largely on the skill level of the group most affected by the virus and whether the costs of HIV/AIDS are financed from savings. If the cost of HIV/AIDS is not financed from savings and the epidemic is concentrated largely among people with lower skill levels, per capita income rises an estimated 0.13–0.17 percent in the worst affected countries. If the cost of HIV/AIDS is financed from savings and the epidemic is concentrated largely among people with higher skill levels, per capita income falls an estimated 0.35–0.60 percent.

An economic growth model currently being developed asserts that other models underestimate the economic impact of HIV/AIDS by not fully capturing the extent and future implications of the destruction of human capital (Bell, Devarajan, and Gersbach 2003). The

Table B2. Summary of Evidence of Macroeconomic Impact of HIV/AIDS

REGION/COUNTRY	IMPACT	AUTHOR	PERIOD
Africa and Sub-Saharan Africa	Annual GDP declines 0.56–1.47 percent. Annual per capita growth is 0.6 percent lower to 0.17 percent higher.	Over (1992)	1990–2025
Sub-Saharan Africa (ordinary least squares and two-stage least squares growth equations)	Economic growth was reduced by 0.8 percent in the 1990s. Annual per capita growth was reduced 1.2 percent between 1990 and 1995.	Bonnel (2000)	1990–97
Tanzania			
Solow-type growth model	Annual GDP growth declines from 3.9 percent without HIV/AIDS to 2.8–3.3 percent. Annual GDP per capita growth declines from 0.7 percent without HIV/AIDS to 0.2–0.7 percent.	Cuddington (1993a)	1985–2010
Solow-type growth model with dual labor market	AIDS reduces real GDP 11–28 percent over period. Per capita income change ranges from increase of 3.6 percent to decrease of 16.1 percent over period.	Cuddington (1993b)	1985–2010
Malawi			
Solow-type growth model	Annual GDP growth rate declines 0.2–1.5 percent. Annual GDP per capita growth declines 0.1–0.3 percent	Cuddington and Hancock (1993a)	1985–2010
Solow-type growth	Annual GDP growth declines 3–9 percent. Annual GDP per capita	Cuddington and	1985–2010

model with dual labor market	growth unchanged or increases by 3 percent.	Hancock (1993b)	1996–2021
Botswana (Cobb-Douglas production function)	Annual GDP growth declines 3.9 percent to 2.0–3.1 percent. After 25 years economy is 24–38 percent smaller. In best-case scenario per capita GDP rises 1.5–1.9 percent a year and average incomes rise 9 percent after 25 years. In worst-case scenario GDP per capita growth declines 1 percent a year and is 13 percent lower after 25 years.	BIDPA (2000)	
South Africa Full supply-demand econometric model	Real GDP falls 0.3 percent lower in 2001, 0.4 percent in 2006–10.	Quattek (2000)	2001–15 (annually through 2005, then 2006–10 and 2011–15)
Computable general equilibrium model	GDP growth decline 2.6 percent in 2008. By 2010 economy is 17 percent smaller, per capita income is 8 percent lower.	Arndt and Lewis (2000)	1997–2010
Trinidad and Tobago, Jamaica	GDP is 4.2 percent lower in Trinidad and Tobago and 6.4 percent lower in Jamaica in 2005.	Nicholls and others (2000)	1997–2005, but results seem to be for 2005

Source: Barnett 2003.

Box B1. The Impact of HIV/AIDS on the Russian Economy

In the absence of strong prevention policies, the number of people in the Russian Federation infected with HIV is expected to increase markedly by 2020 (Ruehl, Pokrovsky, and Vinogradov 2002). Even in the optimistic case (prevalence rate of 1 percent), mortality rates are projected to increase from 500 a month in 2005 to 21,000 a month in 2020, and the cumulative number of people infected with HIV is projected to rise from 1.2 million in 2005 to 2.3 million in 2010 and 5.4 million in 2020.

The pessimistic scenario (prevalence rates of 2–3 percent) results in dramatically higher rates. Under this scenario:

- GDP in 2010 would be as much as 4.15 percent lower than it would have been in the absence of HIV/AIDS; without intervention the loss would rise to 10.5 percent by 2020. Perhaps more significant for long-term development, the uninhibited spread of HIV/AIDS would diminish the economy's long-term growth rate, taking off half a percentage point annually by 2010 and a full percentage point annually by 2020.
- Investment would decline by more than production. Under the pessimistic scenario, investment would fall 5.5 percent in 2010 and 14.5 percent in 2020, creating a severe stumbling block for future growth.
- The effective (that is, quality-adjusted) labor supply would decrease over time, with the overall decline due more to a decline in the number of workers (total labor supply) than to the productivity losses associated with those parts of the work force infected with HIV. This effect reflects the assumption that HIV lowers productivity by a moderate 13 percent.

Using a single-sector growth model, Sharp (2002) concludes that AIDS is likely to have a significant sustained negative impact on aggregate economic growth and annual GDP, with growth falling by 0.2 percent to a little more than 0.5 percent by 2020. Declines in population reduce somewhat the per capita impact at the macroeconomic level.

hypothesis of this model is that by destroying human capital and weakening the transmission of human capital to subsequent generations, HIV/AIDS severely weakens the foundations for economic growth and development. The application of this model to South Africa shows that if nothing is done to combat the epidemic, a complete economic collapse will occur within four generations. If optimal spending on combating the disease and "pooling" (a custom in which children are cared for by extended families) are maintained, growth continues, albeit at a slower pace than in the benchmark case. If pooling breaks down and is replaced by nuclear families, growth will be slower still, even with optimal spending. If school attendance subsidies are not provided, growth will be very sluggish. In all three cases the additional fiscal burden of the interventions is considerable, reinforcing the need for early action to prevent the spread of the epidemic.

Interpretation of the results of the growing number of macroeconomic impact studies being conducted needs to take into account the limitations of such models. Economic modeling is complex, and incorporating an HIV/AIDS scenario requires making assumptions about the rate at which HIV will spread, the number of people infected, their skills and employment, the time from illness to deaths, and the types of care that will be provided. The results depend on the validity of the assumptions. Macro-modeling involves simplification and cannot reflect fully how economies operate in reality. Moreover, to show even small impacts of HIV/AIDS on economic growth, the HIV/AIDS epidemic has to be projected 15–30 years. From the perspective of policymakers struggling with more immediate development challenges, this can reduce the credibility of the impact on economic growth prospects. The potential negative impact of HIV/AIDS on economic growth becomes more real for policymakers when meso and micro impacts of the epidemic—increased government expenditures on treatment and care, increased absenteeism, the costs of replacing skilled labor—are felt at the country level. This tendency reinforces the importance of monitoring and measuring the impact of the epidemic at these levels.

Meso-Level Impacts of HIV/AIDS

HIV/AIDS would have significant impacts at the sectoral level in Eastern Europe and Central Asia.

Health Sector

People with HIV/AIDS have a wide range of health care needs. Some HIV–related conditions can be managed at the primary health care level. As the disease progresses, demands on the health care system change, and care is needed for treatable acute conditions as well as terminal conditions.

As countries adopt HAART, new infrastructure is needed to manage and ensure compliance with complex therapies. If the HIV/AIDS epidemic continues to grow in Eastern Europe and Central Asia, health systems there are likely to face new challenges. These challenges have implications for both public and private health expenditures.

The cost of providing HAART to all people with HIV/AIDS was calculated for each country in Eastern Europe and Central Asia. Based on a low-case (HIV prevalence of 0.50 percent) and a high-case (HIV prevalence of 1 percent) scenario, the number of people with HIV and the number of people with AIDS were calculated.[5] Under the high-case scenario, the number of people with HIV is projected to increase from about 1 million in 2000 to about 5 million in 2010 (figure B1). The number of people with AIDS is projected to increase from 63,000 to about 277,000, while the number of people with tuberculosis is projected to increase from 205,000 to 610,000.

Treatment costs cover treatment for opportunistic infections, diagnostic HIV testing, opportunistic infection prophylaxis, and HAART. Much uncertainty surrounds the future costs of HAART drugs. As a result of the Trade-Related Agreement on Intellectual Property Rights (TRIPS) or local production of HAART drugs (in Brazil and India, for example), the price of HAART has fallen dramatically in many countries. In Eastern Europe and Central Asia,

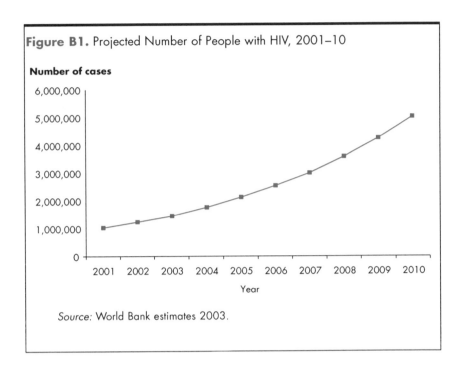

Figure B1. Projected Number of People with HIV, 2001–10

Number of cases

Source: World Bank estimates 2003.

the annual per patient cost of HAART ranges from $200 in Armenia to about $3,600 in Kazakhstan, with an unweighted average of $1,600.[6] Other treatment costs come to $570 per person a year.

A range of treatment costs is used to estimate the potential health expenditures associated with treating people with HIV/AIDS. For low-income countries in the region (that is, countries with per capita GDP of less than $1,200 a year), the lower-range estimates of $970 ($200 for HAART drugs and $570 for other treatment costs) to $2,170 ($1,600 for HAART drugs plus treatment costs and $570 for other treatment costs) are used. For the medium- to high-income countries in the region, estimates of $2,170–$4,170 are used ($3,600 for HAART plus other treatment costs). These ranges are then applied to the low- and high-case scenarios to obtain estimates of health expenditures (table B3). All people with HIV/AIDS are assumed to have access to HAART. It is assumed that each person on HAART will survive two years, during which time treatment will

Table B3. Estimated Costs of Providing HAART to People with HIV/AIDS in the 11 CIS Countries

YEAR	LOW HIV/AIDS SCENARIO		HIGH HIV/AIDS SCENARIO	
	LOW ESTIMATE	HIGH ESTIMATE	LOW ESTIMATE	HIGH ESTIMATE
2001	135,063	260,063	135,063	260,063
2002	155,366,	299,189	155,900	300,244
2003	174,679	336,464	179,417	345,686
2004	191,582	369,193	204,161	393,691
2005	207,716	400,556	233,737	451,213
2006	223,099	430,624	268,969	519,928
2007	237,452	458,887	310,978	602,043
2008	252,197	488,121	361,496	700,975
2009	268,415	520,438	422,891	821,342
2010	285,904	558,547	496,006	964,864
Total	2,131,475	4,122,100	2,619,000	5,049,000

Countries: Armenia, Azerbaijan, Belarus, Georgia, Kazakhstan, Kyrgyz Republic, Republic of Moldova, Russian Federation, Tajikstan, Ukraine, and Uzbekistan.

Source: World Bank estimates 2003.

be provided. This is a conservative estimate, since people on HAART could survive longer, in which case cumulative lifetime HAART costs would be much higher.

By 2010 Eastern European and Central Asian countries will be spending more than $1 billion on HAART, or 1–3 percent of total health expenditures. The bulk of the expenditures will be made by CIS countries such as Kazakhstan, the Russian Federation, and Ukraine. During 1990–98 all Eastern European and Central Asian countries combined spent $60 billion on health care. Potential expenditures on HAART thus do not represent a large percentage of total health care spending, especially when addressed in the context of social or health insurance systems that could effectively pool risks. Health and social insurance systems are still evolving in many Eastern Europe and Central Asia countries, however, and out-of-pocket payments continue to be an important source of health care financing in the region, especially in many low-income CIS countries. Huge disparities exist in annual per capita health care spending, ranging from less than $13 in the poorer Central Asian countries to about $700 in Slovenia (World Bank 2002c).

An optimistic scenario is that by 2010 social insurance systems will be well developed, effectively pooling public and private contributions. A pessimistic scenario is that out-of-pocket payments at the point of service will continue to be a major source of health care financing. In this case treatment costs for HAART are likely to further exacerbate the gap between those who have the ability to pay for treatment and those who do not. More important are concerns about the opportunity cost of public resources for health care and the need to make the best use of available health care resources. Many countries in the region face the challenge of improving health outcomes to achieve levels closer to those in Western Europe. The region's low-income countries, which are facing a combination of communicable and noncommunicable diseases, face very serious resource constraints. Achieving adequate levels of financing for public health programs is a priority in many of these countries. Potential public expenditures on HAART need to be looked at within the broader context of needs, the availability of health care resources, and allocative efficiency concerns. From the perspectives of both public and private financing, a better scenario is to prevent the growth in the number of HIV/AIDS cases through comprehensive prevention programs.

Social Protection

Social protection programs address the needs of vulnerable groups in a society, such as the elderly, children, and the disabled. Premature adult illness and death due to HIV/AIDS will generate important demographic impacts in Eastern Europe and Central Asia. These changes have implications for social protection programs, which are typically funded out of contributions by economically productive age groups and general government revenues.

Based on current demographic indicators, such as total fertility rates, life expectancy, and migration rates, Eastern Europe and Central Asia can be broken into four demographic groups (UNDP 2003):[7]

1. Countries in which the population is aging, most of the population is 20–60, and the birthrate is declining. This group of countries includes Bosnia and Herzegovina; Belarus; Bulgaria; the Czech Republic; Estonia; Georgia; Hungary; Latvia; Lithuania; Macedonia, FYR; Moldova; Poland; Romania; the Russian Federation; Serbia and Montenegro; Slovakia; Slovenia; and Ukraine.

2. Countries in which birthrates are high, life expectancy low, and the population young. This group of countries includes Tajikistan, Turkmenistan, and Uzbekistan.

3. Countries in which the population is older than in the first two groups and there are fewer children, due to falling birthrates. This group of countries includes Azerbaijan, Kazakhstan, and the Kyrgyz Republic.

4. A residual group of countries that includes Albania and Armenia.

The first group of countries includes all of the countries in the region in which HIV/AIDS is spreading fastest (Belarus, Estonia, Latvia, Moldova, the Russian Federation, and Ukraine). The high prevalence of HIV/AIDS in countries with declining fertility is an indication of the possible future demographic impact of the epidemic. The dependency ratio in these countries is likely to increase as a result of premature mortality. For example, by 2015 the Russian Federation is projected to have just four workers for every three nonworkers. Changes in the dependency ratio in Russia will affect social security and pensions (Sharp 2002).

In the second group of countries, where total fertility rates are still at replacement levels, the HIV/AIDS epidemic has the potential to increase the number of orphans. Orphans face a bleak future, and providing for them will greatly increase the costs of social protection programs.

In the third group of countries, the combination of elderly people and children under 15 will generate substantial social protection needs in the short to medium terms. In addition, social protection programs will most likely have to be expanded to include home or community-based care for people with AIDS.

Firm-Level Impacts

The spread of HIV/AIDS affects industry and commerce. For firms to earn a profit, the total cost of production has to be less than total revenues. Production costs are a function of inputs, such as labor, materials, and utilities. The increased prevalence of HIV/AIDS raises the costs of doing business by increasing labor costs. Specific effects include the following (Barnett and Whiteside 2002):

- Absenteeism increases among employees who are sick or who take time off to care for sick family members.

- Worker productivity falls.

- Labor turnover is high, as sick employees take early retirement or die. Firms bear additional costs associated with training new staff.

- Firms need to maintain a larger workforce on their payrolls as a contingency measure and to maintain production schedules.

- As skilled workers become scarce, the wages of remaining workers may rise.

- The business environment may change, with investors reluctant to commit funds if they think HIV/AIDS and its impact will compromise their investments and returns.

Only a few studies have been conducted on the impact of HIV/AIDS on firms, most of them concentrated in Southern Africa, particularly South Africa. These studies show that one of the most critical problems faced by firms in countries with high HIV/AIDS prevalence is absenteeism, which can increase labor costs 37 percent. Fifteen percent of absenteeism is attributable to HIV/AIDS (Roberts, Rau, and Emery 1996). Another major source of increased costs are the benefits that have to be paid to workers with HIV/AIDS—a lump-sum payment upon death, a pension to the surviving spouse, and a disability pension. These benefits accounted for 7 percent of payroll costs in 2001. By 2010 they are projected to rise to 18 percent.

The firm-level impacts of HIV/AIDS could have serious implications for Eastern European and Central Asian countries, many of which are emerging markets. A World Bank report (2002f) notes the key role of the entry and growth of new firms—especially small and medium-size enterprises—in generating economic growth and creating employment. In the next 10 years, the World Bank will be encouraging countries that are lagging behind in the development of new firms, especially small and medium-size enterprises, to focus on this issue and improve the environment for their entry and development. Among this group are most of the CIS countries in which HIV infection rates are rapidly increasing, including Belarus, the Russian Federation, and Ukraine. In encouraging the development of new firms, however, the continued growth of the HIV/AIDS epidemic needs to be taken into account. A rapid rise in HIV/AIDS in the generalized population could seriously threaten the ability of new private firms, especially small and medium-size enterprises, to survive in an increasingly competitive environment.

Impact on Households

HIV/AIDS can have a profound effect on households. The death of a breadwinner can cause a household to face a shock in terms of its daily sustenance. It can cause older children to drop out of school to join the labor force and younger children to take on new household duties, including caring for younger siblings. Dropping out of formal education can have serious intergenerational impacts on the household, essentially relegating it to a lower socioeconomic status than it might have had if the breadwinner had not died. Where multiple members of the household are infected with HIV, the household may disintegrate and disappear. There are methodological challenges to identifying these disappeared households, which makes it difficult to measure this dimension of household impact.

The impact of HIV/AIDS is also felt in terms of changes in household composition and structure. In countries with high prevalence, new forms of households have emerged after people between 15 and 45 die. These include households with elderly household heads with young children (usually their grandchildren), large households with unrelated foster or orphaned children, households headed by children, and single-parent households. Some evidence suggests that these new forms of households are not as efficient as traditional households and are highly susceptible to poverty and deprivation (Shell 2000).

The limited evidence on the impact of HIV/AIDS on household expenditures and consumption suggests that the share of food and nonfood expenditures changes. Households in which an adult dies spend 33 percent less on nonfood items such as clothing, soap, and batteries, and their food purchases decrease as well (Ainsworth, Frasen, and Over 1998).

A household survey in Thailand found that out-of-pocket medical care for people with HIV/AIDS equals about six months of average total household income (Pitayanon, Kongsin, and Janjareon 2000). However, the largest economic cost of an HIV/AIDS–related death is forgone earnings, which are higher than average for people who die of AIDS because they die earlier. Taking care of a person with HIV/AIDS also affects the household labor supply.

Poverty, Inequality, and Human Development Impacts

The impact of HIV/AIDS on poverty can be looked at from a macro or a micro perspective. At the macro level, changes in the Gini coefficient are an important measure of the impact on poverty and inequality. There is little evidence of these impacts. However, it has been hypothesized that HIV/AIDS has the potential to exacerbate inequality, since certain groups have better access to health care services than others. Better-off groups are able to afford antiretroviral drug therapy, thereby reducing the negative health effects and disability associated with full-blown AIDS. In contrast, poor households are not able to afford antiretroviral drugs or treatment for opportunistic infections. These differences have welfare implications for households.

In many countries (South Africa, Thailand, the United States), the HIV/AIDS epidemic was initially concentrated among the wealthy and the better educated. As the epidemic matured, it tended to concentrate among low-income groups. This shift in the concentration of the epidemic has implications at the intercountry and intracountry levels. It has been hypothesized that over time HIV/AIDS will become more closely associated with poverty and increase the vulnerability of countries and groups within countries to poverty, potentially exacerbating the "poverty trap" (Bloom and Jaypee 2002).

Health is an important nonincome dimension of poverty. Insofar as HIV/AIDS affects health and well-being and reduces human capability, it increases poverty. However, to understand the impact of HIV/AIDS on poverty, it is necessary to compare its health impacts with those of other highly prevalent diseases in a country. No known studies have attempted to compare HIV/AIDS with other diseases using comparable measures, such as DALYs or quality-adjusted life years (QALYs).

The Costs of Delaying Action

Countries faced with the potentially rapid spread of HIV/AIDS have two options: delay HIV/AIDS interventions while prevalence rates are still low and intervene only once the HIV/AIDS epidemic has become visible, or implement comprehensive prevention and treatment programs early on while prevalence rates are still low (Bonnel 2000). Cost-benefit and cost-effectiveness analyses of HIV/AIDS programs can help policymakers make informed decisions about resource allocation. By measuring and comparing the costs and consequences of different interventions, they can evaluate the relative efficiency of these interventions and estimate resource requirements. Cost-benefit analysis measures consequences in monetary terms and requires analysts to make decisions about the monetary value to be attached to, for example, an AIDS death. In cost-effectiveness analysis such value judgments are not required, and consequences are measured in terms of infections or deaths averted.

Cost-benefit analysis of HIV/AIDS programs for all Eastern European and Central Asian countries was conducted for 2001–10. For each country the costs of implementing a comprehensive prevention program were obtained and assumptions made about coverage rates and population risk groups. The cost, population, and coverage data were derived from estimates by the U.N. General Assembly Special Session on AIDS (UNGASS) for global HIV/AIDS program resource needs, which were then refined for countries in the region (Schwartlander and others 2001b). The number of HIV/AIDS infections averted as a result of implementing prevention programs was calculated using the AIDS Impact Model (AIMS).[8] The direct benefits of HIV prevention programs are saved lives, prevented disease, avoided or diminished disability, reduced absenteeism, and saved treatment costs. These benefits can be converted into monetary terms and compared with program costs to derive net benefits (benefits net of investments in prevention). Direct costs refer to the costs of treating people with HIV/AIDS; indirect costs refer to the averted costs from an AIDS death measured in terms of productive life years and wages. Costs minus benefits (both measured in dollar terms) produce net benefits. Since a dollar earned in the future is less valuable than a dollar earned in the present, all future net benefits are discounted, at a rate of 10 percent.

Comparison of the costs of prevention programs and economic benefits shows that benefits from averted HIV infections far exceed the costs. Cost-benefit analyses of HIV/AIDS prevention programs in the Russian Federation, for example, show that net benefits are potentially large, with the benefit-cost ratio clearly in favor of prevention (table B4). Governments in Eastern Europe and Central Asia would thus be well served by adopting HIV/AIDS prevention programs early.

Table B4. Cost-Benefit Analysis of HIV/AIDS Prevention Programs in the Russian Federation, 2001–10
(current dollars)

YEAR	COSTS OF INTERVENTION	DIRECT BENEFITS	INDIRECT BENEFITS	TOTAL BENEFITS	NET BENEFITS	TOTAL BENEFITS
2001	0	0	0	0	0	0
2002	0	0	0	0	0	0
2003	85,784	0	0	0	–85,784	–85,784
2004	100,271	0	0	0	–100,271	–100,271
2005	115,174	33,689	1,034,849	1,068,538	953,364	787,904
2006	131,082	58,286	2,032,935	2,091,221	1,960,139	1,472,681
2007	150,001	92,356	3,458,975	3,551,331	3,401,330	2,323,154
2008	168,001	135,549	5,435243	5,570,792	5,402,791	3,354,708
2009	188,161	189,976	7,937,567	8,127,542	7,939,381	4,481,574
2010	225,793	256,401	11,083,955	11,340,355	11,114,562	5,703,527

Source: World Bank Estimates 2003.

Conclusion

The potential economic and social impacts of a generalized HIV/AIDS epidemic in Eastern Europe and Central Asia are large. In the case of a generalized epidemic causing premature illness and death in the productive age groups, the following impacts are possible:

• Economic growth rates could decline by 0.5–1.0 percentage points a year.

• Health expenditures for treating people with HIV/AIDS could increase 1–3 percent. These expenditures could be effectively addressed through social and health insurance systems. However, evidence from many Eastern Europe and Central Asia countries, particularly the CIS countries, shows that social insurance systems are still evolving. In several countries, especially the low-income CIS countries, out-of-pocket spending is one of the most important sources of health care financing. There is a risk that expenditures for HAART would be borne by households, contributing to a growing gap in health status between different income groups in society. Potential public expenditures on HAART need to be looked at in the broader context of health care needs, the availability of resources, and allocative efficiency concerns. Both in terms of potential public and private spending on HAART, a better option is to invest now in averting new infections.

- The dependency ratio could change, putting strain on social protection systems, especially in countries already experiencing declining fertility rates (Belarus, Estonia, Moldova, the Russian Federation).

- Household size and composition could change, with an increase in single-parent households, households managed by the elderly, and households headed by children. This change could exacerbate the vulnerability of households, with negative intergenerational effects on households as children are forced to drop out of school to work or take care of siblings, thereby reinforcing the "poverty trap."

Estimates of the costs and benefits of prevention programs clearly show that the benefits associated with prevention programs outweigh program costs. Countries thus need to emphasize prevention as part of a program that also includes treatment.

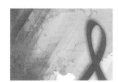

ANNEX C

Interventions against HIV/AIDS and Tuberculosis in Eastern Europe and Central Asia: The Evidence Base and Gaps in Knowledge

This annex reviews the evidence on the effectiveness of interventions against HIV/AIDS and tuberculosis, primarily at the population level. It draws on examples and lessons learned globally while focusing on Eastern Europe and Central Asia. Because HIV prevalence rates are low throughout the region (with the exception of high-prevalence pockets, such as St. Petersburg, Russia), the discussion emphasizes prevention efforts. Most of these rely on population-based and multisectoral public health approaches, including surveillance, education, evaluation, and data-based policy implementation.

Prevention Strategies

In many countries in the region, the overall prevalence of HIV is low but rates are high among vulnerable subgroups, such as injecting drug users, commercial sex workers, and, to a much smaller extent, men who have sex with men. Even where HIV prevalence is low in vulnerable subpopulations, other sexually transmitted infections and high-risk behaviors, such as sharing needles, may be common, signaling that HIV prevalence may increase in the future. In most countries, therefore, there is a historical opportunity to prevent the potential explosion of HIV infection. It is often difficult to mobilize the necessary political commitment in a low-prevalence setting. The prevention approach thus necessitates calling attention to the history of other countries in which prevalence was low in the early stages of the epidemic and exploded due to widespread precursor risks and inaction.

Given this low prevalence in most of the region, understanding the efficacy and cost-effectiveness of prevention efforts is critical to the efficient use of scarce health system resources. It may take considerable time for prevalence to increase to high levels in the region, but low prevalence does not justify complacency: if each infected person transmits HIV to more than one other person on average, the epidemic will inevitably grow. If the precursor social and behavioral conditions to the spread of HIV are recognized, this growth can be abated. In Eastern Europe and Central Asia, such precursors are evident.

Poverty, the degradation of national health systems, and postconflict and post-Soviet social disruption have created vulnerabilities and risk conditions in the region. This section examines public health approaches to these risk conditions and to prevention practices, considering the broader social context and the need for a multisectoral approach.[9] It does not focus on interventions targeting people already infected with HIV, except as these interventions can prevent the spread of HIV from them.

To better understand the concept of prevention in the context of the HIV/AIDS epidemic in the region, it is helpful to review the theoretical bases for prevention science. Three stages of prevention can be distinguished:

- Primary prevention refers to interventions applied before infection or onset of disease. Examples include treatment of sexually transmitted infections other than HIV, condom use to protect uninfected people, and school-based education about the risk factors associated with HIV transmission.

- Secondary prevention refers to interventions applied after the acquisition of the virus but before the onset of symptomatic illness. Interventions include HAART, which delays the progression from HIV infection to AIDS and may prevent transmission to others by lowering the potential of the carrier to infect others (an example of primary prevention for the individual yet to be infected). An example of secondary prevention of syphilis would be treatment of primary syphilis in order to prevent progression to secondary syphilis.

- Tertiary prevention refers to interventions applied after a disease has been contracted but before significant disability has occurred. After the onset of AIDS, tertiary prevention may include social services and palliative care to prevent destitution and physical suffering experienced in the end stages of AIDS.

Many modes of primary HIV prevention exist, the efficacy of which may vary by country. In the low-prevalence nations of Eastern Europe and Central Asia, broad-based population approaches alone will not be as cost-effective as approaches focusing on highly vulnerable groups (Brown and others 2001; Walker 2003). It is also important to target not only particular risk groups but also their sex partners and sexual networks.

Strategies developed in other regions to prevent the spread of HIV include:

- Blood screening and promotion of blood safety.

- Mass media campaigns.

- Educational projects targeting young people.

- Social marketing of condoms.

- Treatment of sexually transmitted infections.

- Educational projects targeting commercial sex workers and their clients.

- Harm reduction strategies among injecting drug users.

- Voluntary counseling and testing.

- Prevention of mother-to-child transmission.

- Use of microbicides and female-controlled methods for preventing sexually transmitted diseases.

The appropriate mix of primary prevention strategies can be effective in changing risk behavior and subsequently HIV transmission in low- and middle-income countries (Merson, Dayton, and O'Reilly 2000). If applied early enough, primary prevention techniques can even significantly reduce the national prevalence of HIV/AIDS in more well-established epidemics. However, little evidence has been compiled on the relative cost and likely impact of different interventions in Eastern Europe and Central Asia.

Infrastructure for HIV prevention is needed as part of health system development. So, too, are development efforts in other sectors, such as labor, military, education, and civil society. Creation of this infrastructure requires identification of risk groups, surveillance of trends of infection within these subpopulations, assessment of behaviors leading to the spread of HIV, and surveillance of risk factors such as injecting drug use (particularly needle sharing), sexually transmitted infection incidence and treatment, and sexual practices associated with HIV/AIDS. In low-prevalence countries, behavioral change may be the most important primary prevention channel. Thus behavioral surveillance, especially among vulnerable subpopulations, is an important surveillance need. Without clear identification of patterns of risk behavior, monitoring of behavior change in response to education and policy interventions, and development of knowledge on risk group behaviors in general, primary prevention efforts cannot be scientifically applied.

In Eastern Europe and Central Asia, health system projects funded by the World Bank often address reforms in terms of financing, rationalizing, and increasing access to packages of services. In a multisectoral approach, improving public health requires expanded thinking to ensure financing for public goods (such as surveillance systems and clinical trials specific to pilot projects among high-risk groups) that might not be included in financing packages for direct medical care services. Promoting health, tracing and testing contacts of high-risk people, and addressing marginalized populations' needs have not been prominent in health systems projects. Sometimes this may mean adding specific components to address public health infrastructure; in other cases it may mean providing for specific training and technical assistance in the fields of HIV/AIDS and tuberculosis control.

Surveillance

Effective surveillance systems are key to controlling any infectious disease, but HIV surveillance systems need to be tailored to the state of the epidemic (Schwartlander, Ghys, and others 2001). In low-level and concentrated settings, doing so requires focusing on monitoring key population subgroups with higher risk levels rather than general population groups, such as prenatal clinic attendees (Brown and others 2001). Surveillance data can also be used to mobilize public opinion and to monitor the success of a government's or community's response to an epidemic in terms of observing both behavior change and changes in sero-prevalence.

In Eastern Europe and Central Asia, very little is known about the true extent of the epidemic or the response of various risk populations to any of the interventions undertaken to date (Hamers and Downs 2003; Novotny, Haazen, and Adeyi 2003). Data on newly diagnosed HIV infections depend on patterns of HIV testing and reporting, and coverage in Eastern Europe and Central Asia is very incomplete (EuroHIV 2002). There is little evidence, for example, of the spread of HIV among men who have sex with men in the region, although this lack of evidence probably reflects the marginalization of this subgroup rather than the low level of sero-prevalence.

Biological surveillance is a key element for planning and assessing primary and secondary prevention activities. This type of surveillance includes:

- Ongoing HIV screening of donated blood, which also serves as a tool for eliminating the spread of HIV through blood transfusion.

- Sentinel serological surveillance of defined risk group subpopulations (such as injecting drug users, commercial sex workers, mobile populations). This type of surveillance can be done through special clinics, treatment facilities for injecting drug users, sexually transmitted infection clinics, and employment sites.

- Anonymous HIV testing of blood samples of specimens taken from general population surveys used for other purposes (blood lead screening, cholesterol levels, and so forth). If a demographic and health survey that includes blood sampling is undertaken, sera could be submitted for HIV screening as anonymous, unlinked specimens.

- Anonymous or nonanonymous HIV screening of specimens taken as part of special population surveys (as in research or evaluation studies).

- Anonymous or nonanonymous HIV testing of people using voluntary counseling and testing sites.

Limitations exist in each of these serological access points. The sensitivity and specificity of laboratory tests are important, because in low-prevalence settings, even with highly sensitive tests, the predictive value of such tests is very limited.[10] Thus screening in Eastern Europe and Central Asia should be limited to people with high-risk profiles. Given the limited, passive surveillance systems now in place, most of the high-risk groups will not be screened. However, with a broader collection of serologic data, these disparate sources can provide a broad picture of the epidemic in a region or country.

In Western Europe the most frequently used methods of population screening for HIV include sampling pregnant women, testing blood donors, and testing drug users and people with sexually transmitted infections who volunteer to be tested (Hamers and others 2003). Beginning in 1999 some sentinel surveillance activities of commercial sex workers and men who have sex with men were implemented in Eastern Europe and Central Asia, but these activities have not been integrated into national program activities to monitor HIV/AIDS epidemics. Because of low utilization, little useful population-based information has come from anonymous voluntary counseling and testing sites (Grund 2001; Dehne and others 2000). Data based on diagnostic testing from referral hospitals and specialty clinics are subject to significant participation bias because of the stigmatization associated with HIV infection and the nonrepresentative nature of such data collection.

Sentinel surveillance may track infection in subpopulations by drawing blood for other diagnostic purposes or during routine check-ups. It can either be stripped of identifying markers to ensure anonymity and minimal bias or reported back to the patient (together with pre- and posttest counseling). When samples are purposefully collected for HIV testing, informed consent is necessary. Positive test results require referral and possible treatment, which may not be available in all health systems in the region. With informed consent comes participation bias: people who do not wish to know their HIV status or have it reported will not be tested.

Another area in critical need of improvement is behavioral surveillance. Good cross-sectional behavioral surveillance data will identify subpopulations at risk and help focus serological sampling efforts to yield maximum population information. Behavioral surveillance can identify risk behaviors associated with HIV transmission in both the general population and subpopulations, such as vulnerable young people, to help target future prevention interventions. National and risk group–targeted surveys include questions on behaviors that lead to risk (sharing needles, not using condoms, trading sex for drugs), as well as questions about attitudes and knowledge of transmission methods and prevention practices.

In order to tailor behavioral surveillance systems to specific epidemic conditions, it may be useful to consider several key questions posed by Pisani (2002) regarding low-level and concentrated epidemics such as found in Eastern Europe and Central Asia:

• Are there risk behaviors that might lead to an HIV epidemic?

- In which subpopulations are those behaviors concentrated?

- How common are the risk behaviors?

- How large are these subpopulations?

- How high is HIV prevalence in these subpopulations?

- What are the links between subpopulations?

Behavioral surveillance is seldom integrated into national surveillance programs for HIV/AIDS, but reports have shown the value of such information. A study of 239 injecting drug users recruited from community sites in St. Petersburg reported that 41 percent regularly shared needles, most had multiple sexual partners, and 70 percent engaged in intercourse without condoms (Somlai and others 2002). Given the high rates of syphilis and other sexually transmitted infections in St. Petersburg, the potential for transmission among bridge populations is enormous.

Reported behavioral indicators of risk include (Pisani 2002):

- Having had sex with a nonregular partner in the past 12 months.

- Not having used a condom during last sexual contact with a nonregular partner.

- Having early onset of sexual activity (younger than age 13).

- Sharing unclean injecting equipment.

- Having multiple sexual partners (injecting drug users).

- Having large number of clients per week, irregularly using condoms, and having poor access to condoms (for commercial sex workers).

- Being highly mobile.

Reporting of HIV/AIDS cases to the WHO and the EuroHIV Centre, required of all countries, may represent only a population-based assessment of the tertiary disease burden (that is, full-blown

AIDS rather than HIV sero-positivity among vulnerable or general populations). HIV/AIDS data include reporting country, age at diagnosis, gender, date of diagnosis, date of report, transmission category, HIV/AIDS indicative diseases at diagnosis, type of virus, date of first HIV–positive test, vital status (alive or deceased), and date of death. Reporting of AIDS cases does not, however, adequately convey the nature and rapidly changing dynamics of the HIV epidemic. The number of people with AIDS increases only years after HIV incidence rates increase.

Forty-one countries in the European Region of the WHO had nationwide reporting systems for HIV by the end of 2000. Data through the end of 2001 indicate that rates of HIV infection have increased much more rapidly rate in Eastern Europe than in Western or Central Europe. The largest increases were in the Russian Federation (374 per million), Estonia (276 per million), and Latvia (195 per million) (Hamers and Downs 2003). While heterosexual transmission has increased in the region, infection by injecting drug users remains the main source of new reported infections. Thus behavioral and sentinel biologic surveillance among injecting drug users is critical to understanding the HIV/AIDS epidemic in the region. Although efforts are currently being made to improve both biological and behavioral surveillance in the region (surveys in major cities in the Russian Federation were conducted by the Vozrastcheniye Foundation and the Research Institute for Complex Social Studies of the St. Petersburg State University in 1997–98, for example [Smolskaya 1999]), additional targeted efforts are needed.

Evidence suggests that both Uganda and Thailand have improved intervention programs based on the results of behavioral and biological surveillance. In Thailand, where surveillance of HIV/AIDS is comprehensive, data from population-based behavioral surveys showed that about 25 percent of all men visited commercial sex workers; sentinel serologic surveillance data indicated that 44 percent of commercial sex workers in Chiang Mai were infected with HIV (WHO and others 2000). Publication of these data encouraged the development of a 100 percent condom use policy for brothels; implementation of broad-based public education about HIV/AIDS risks; involvement of multiple other sectors of society, such as media, transportation, and labor; and development of human rights protections for infected people. The incidence of HIV infection in Thailand fell 80 percent from the level reported before implementation of the national program (USAID and the Synergy Project 2002).

In Uganda sentinel sites showed a significant decline in incidence after high-level political support was declared by the President of Uganda and multisectoral responses were supported, including responses by the education, transportation, entertainment, and media sectors (USAID and the Synergy Project 2002). Without appropriate sentinel surveillance, linkage of program efforts to outcomes might not have been possible.

Other sources of information for HIV surveillance include tracking death registration, behavioral studies, and sexually transmitted infection data (which reveal unprotected sex outside of monogamous relationships). The results of syphilis testing among pregnant women, for example, may be a part of HIV surveillance systems if used as an indicator of risk behavior. Surveillance of other conditions, such as hepatitis B and C and tuberculosis, can also be used to indicate population risks for HIV infection. The new surveillance system for sexually transmitted diseases being implemented across Europe will improve public health tracking of sexual behavior indicators (Hamers and Downs 2003).

Newer techniques, such as rapid HIV testing using non-laboratory-based methodologies (OraQuick HIV rapid test [U.S. CDC 2003a]), could improve the ability to conduct surveillance, particularly in difficult to reach populations (Phili and Vardas 2002). These techniques do not depend on referral to specialist clinics and laboratories or on later follow-up for feedback of results They do, however, depend on outreach by trained testers and counselors and on the availability of referral mechanisms for people who test positive. They provide patients with their results immediately, so that they may be encouraged to refer their sex partners (and needle-sharing partners) for testing and be encouraged to change their risk behavior to prevent the spread of HIV.

Surveillance data can generate a public response to the HIV epidemic, especially in regions where it is still invisible. Identifying the links between risk groups and the general population is critical to understanding the nature of HIV/AIDS epidemics in the region. In addition, it is important to understand the beliefs and attitudes of health care professionals and political decisionmakers who can shape national responses to HIV/AIDS.

Given the evidence that surveillance systems in other regions have been an important tool for tracking and identifying the course of the HIV epidemic, the World Bank will encourage efforts to improve public health infrastructure as part of health system reform. Specific HIV/AIDS surveillance indicators should be incorporated into any new health information system programs at their inception (Hamers and others 2003). The World Bank's comparative advantage in this area is in supporting public health surveillance system development as part of overall health systems operations and broader disease prevention programs. It could support operational research to understand the bridging between risk groups and general populations, to evaluate specific program applications among high-risk groups, and to inform dialogue with decisionmakers across disciplines and levels of government to ensure leadership on the prevention of HIV/AIDS in Eastern Europe and Central Asia.

Table C1 summarizes the specific key objectives, target groups, methods, and possible priorities for developing HIV/AIDS surveillance systems in the region. The World Bank's comparative advantage in each of these areas will vary from country to country, depending on the most important risk groups, the status of the epidemic, the technical capacity of the client country, and cooperation with partner agencies.

Voluntary Counseling and Testing

The crucial role of voluntary counseling and testing has been recognized in Sub-Saharan Africa and Southeast Asia, the regions hardest hit by the HIV/AIDS epidemic. Voluntary counseling and testing are of paramount importance in both preventing and treating

HIV/AIDS. This process involves pretest counseling, posttest counseling, and biologic testing for the presence of HIV antibodies, usually by blood or saliva. In addition to testing for the presence of HIV, this intervention, usually performed by a specially trained health educator or counselor, helps identify risk behaviors that should be changed to prevent further transmission, encourages sex and needle-sharing partners to be tested for HIV, and provides information about services for people infected with HIV (including possible treatment). This process is often anonymous, but when conducted as a referral to a specialty hospital—the usual pattern in Eastern Europe and Central Asia—this is not always the case. Depending on the resources of the clinic or testing center, participants may receive their results immediately or they may have to return in several days to receive their results. Not surprisingly, most people express a strong preference for receiving their results immediately (Respess, Rayfield, and Dondero 2001). Newer, faster testing technology may increase utilization of voluntary counseling and testing.

Voluntary counseling and testing in Eastern Europe and Central Asia is usually not provided in stand-alone centers. Instead, this intervention is usually provided by general hospitals or clinics, typically within the reproductive health or infectious disease departments. These services are also provided by NGO–based clinical projects facilities such as Médicins Sans Frontières, the Open Society Institute, and the International Committee of the Red Cross. Novel approaches to providing this service include mobile testing services in rural communities, in places where drug users congregate, in places where commercial sex workers are active, and in populations groups with marginal medical care (for example, in Roma communities). Mobile outreach work, including referral to voluntary counseling and testing, has been conducted in Bulgaria, along with needle exchange and education, but the outcomes have not yet been evaluated. Participants are counseled on various strategies to inform their sexual partners of their status and to encourage them to be tested.

Several potential positive outcomes result from participating in voluntary counseling and testing services, but there is a significant risk that identification of HIV status among already highly stigma-

Table C1. Objectives, Target Groups, and Methods for HIV/AIDS Surveillance in Eastern Europe and Central Asia

SURVEILLANCE OBJECTIVE	TARGET GROUP	METHOD	PRIORITY/ TIMING
Risk behavior in vulnerable groups	Injecting drug users, commercial sex workers, young people, mobile populations	Cross-sectional surveys among target groups	1
Knowledge among young people	Out-of-school young people, students, military recruits	School-based behavioral surveys; special research for out-of-school young people	2
Knowledge/attitudes among health professionals	Physicians, health policymakers, insurance program managers	Special research studies	1
Population behavioral and sero-prevalence (bridge population)	Pregnant women, general population	Prenatal clinic blood sampling, blood sampling and questions from demographic and health surveys	4
Risk group sero-prevalence	Injecting drug users, commercial sex workers, mobile populations, military personnel, patients of sexually transmitted infection clinics	Inclusion of HIV testing on specimens, work with NGOs for access	2
Serological trends over time in risk groups	Injecting drug users, commercial sex workers, mobile populations, military personnel, patients of sexually transmitted infection clinics	Inclusion of HIV testing on specimens, work with NGOs for access	4
Virologic resistance and subtypes	All people tested	Any specimen referred for HIV testing	5
Program evaluation	Injecting drug users, commercial sex workers, mobile populations, military personnel, patients of sexually transmitted infection clinics	Any specimen referred for HIV testing	4

Note: 1 = now, high priority; 2 = soon, high priority; 3 = soon, medium priority; 4 = future, medium priority; 5 = future, low priority.
Source: World Bank.

tized populations will lead to job loss, social disruption, and increased marginalization. Testing can help alter the risk behavior of those who test negative, however, improving their chances of remaining so. In low-prevalence countries, people may not feel comfortable visiting stand-alone voluntary counseling and testing centers for fear of being identified as at risk for HIV. For this reason, where appropriate, voluntary counseling and testing services may need to be further integrated into health service activities, by including HIV testing as a routine part of medical care when indicated by the risk profile of the patient population. Simplified HIV–testing procedures (rapid diagnostic tests) may also be applied. Such procedures are part of a new HIV/AIDS initiative now under evaluation by the Centers for Disease Control and Prevention in the United States (U.S. CDC 2003a). Voluntary counseling and testing should be seen as a gateway to services rather than simply a surveillance or information collection tool.

Clinical trials in Kenya, Tanzania, and Trinidad demonstrated the cost-effectiveness of voluntary counseling and testing in reducing HIV risk behavior (Coates 2000; Walker 2003). Similar results were found in a voluntary counseling and testing program in Rwanda (Allen and others 1992). Results from Uganda highlight the link between voluntary counseling and testing and changes in risk behavior. After the widespread introduction of voluntary counseling and testing in 1990, condom use rose from 10 percent to 89 percent with steady partners and from 28 percent to 100 percent with non-steady partners within several years of program implementation (USAID and Synergy Project 2002). Similar findings have been documented in the United States, where anonymous testing has been linked to earlier medical treatment for people with HIV and reductions in HIV risk behavior (Valdiserri and others 2000).

In most of Eastern Europe and Central Asia, there is a need to increase public awareness of the availability of voluntary counseling and testing and to diversify the locations of testing centers. Goodwin and others (2003) report that 40 percent of a sample of people from business communities in Georgia and Poland did not know where they could be tested for HIV.

Further complicating the implementation of targeted voluntary counseling and testing in Eastern Europe is the history of testing in the region. Bulgaria and the Russian Federation had compulsory testing in the early 1990s, which served to identify people with HIV as "social deviants." Discrimination against people with the disease persists today (Rhodes and others 1999).

The lack of testing facilities, the lack of culturally appropriate approaches to testing, and the general public's limited knowledge about HIV are all barriers to voluntary counseling and testing. These issues need to be addressed if voluntary counseling and testing is to become an effective intervention in the region, particularly among high-risk groups. In countries with high prevalence rates, there is strong evidence that voluntary counseling and testing can have a positive impact on changing high-risk behavior and that informing people of their HIV status is useful. In countries with low-level and concentrated epidemics, where appropriate, voluntary counseling and testing services could be incorporated into general health centers and special facilities for marginalized groups, not provided at stand-alone testing centers. In addition, public information about the availability of voluntary counseling and testing for those at high risk may need to be socially marketed in order to educate both the groups themselves and the general public about its availability and appropriateness (Global HIV Prevention Working Group 2002). This does not mean that everyone in Eastern Europe and Central Asia should be tested; resources are insufficient for this inefficient and cost-ineffective approach. Voluntary counseling and testing should target high-risk groups, and the barriers for voluntary counseling and testing among these groups should be addressed.

Voluntary counseling and testing can also be used in conjunction with National Tuberculosis Program activities. In 1998 the WHO launched the ProTEST initiative, to set up operational links between HIV prevention and control and National Tuberculosis Program or general health services. The initiative involves both provision of and demand for voluntary counseling and testing for HIV as entry points to a range of HIV and tuberculosis prevention and care interventions. In addition to voluntary counseling and testing, the range of services provided under ProTEST includes tuberculosis screening and active case finding, treatment of active cases, secondary and tertiary preventive interventions for people with HIV or AIDS, treatment of sexually transmitted diseases, and support and care for people with HIV/AIDS. The initiative is still experimental in a few countries in Sub-Saharan Africa; national coverage is expected in three to five years (http://www.who.int/gtb/policyrd/TBHIV.htm#ProTEST). Preliminary cost-effectiveness analyses indicate that voluntary counseling and testing, and the subsequent treatment of active cases or preventive therapy, are relatively affordable (http://www.who.int/gtb/tuberculosisHIV/Durban_feb03/index.htm).

The World Bank's comparative advantage in this intervention lies in its capacity for multisectoral policy dialogue concerning the high-risk groups who bridge to the larger population. Increased availability of voluntary counseling and testing through targeted approaches can be integrated into multisectoral and health system operations supported by the Bank.

Harm Reduction Strategies

Injecting drug use was not widespread before the fall of the Soviet Union. In fact, draconian police policies probably had a great deal of impact in preventing drug trafficking in the Soviet Union (Kelly and Amirkhanian 2003).

Studies of injecting drug users in Southeast Asia provide clear evidence of the risk for the explosive spread of HIV associated with such groups (USAID and the Synergy Project 2002). HIV transmission through commercial sex workers in Southeast Asia has been attenuated through 100 percent condom use in brothels, but the epidemic among injecting drug users continues unabated.

The populations of commercial sex workers and injecting drug users overlap significantly. Western countries have reported little success in controlling the HIV epidemic among injecting drug users through supply-side drug interdiction modalities. However, supply-side interventions in Eastern Europe and Central Asia may require further investigation; as yet, little investigation of such interventions has been undertaken. Given the youth, mobility, and behavioral patterns supporting spread to bridge populations of injecting drugs users, it is unlikely that the HIV epidemic will remain confined to this group (Kelly and Amirkhanian 2003).

Harm reduction is a somewhat controversial approach to reducing risk among subpopulations, primarily injecting drug users and commercial sex workers. It recognizes that drug treatment programs rarely attain total abstinence and that the number of commercial sex workers will expand in the face of economic deprivation in Eastern Europe and Central Asia (Singer 1997; Open Society Institute and International Harm Reduction Development 2002). This approach promotes programs that minimize or reduce transmission in the face of persistent risk behavior, lowering but not eliminating risk. Harm reduction programs include needle and syringe exchanges, drug dependency treatment and rehabilitation, and 100 percent condom use programs for commercial sex workers.

In New York City an advanced epidemic among injecting drug users was reversed through legal, widespread needle and syringe exchange programs; counseling; testing; and outreach activities (Des Jarlais and others 1996, 2000). Between 1991 and 1996 HIV incidence among injecting drug users declined more than 40 percent. Needle and syringe exchange programs are often linked to other services, thus providing a bridge to HIV/AIDS information, risk reduction materials (bleach and condoms), voluntary counseling and testing, and referrals to drug abuse treatment and other social services (Global HIV Prevention Working Group 2002).

Little is known about behaviors among injecting drug users in Eastern Europe and Central Asia, and there have been no rigorous evaluation studies of harm reduction programs provided to this subpopulation. It is likely that harm reduction programs for injecting drug users are cost-effective, though. In Belarus, for example, the cost of averting a single HIV infection was estimated at $68 (UNAIDS 2000).

Most needle and syringe exchange programs in Eastern Europe and Central Asia are conducted by local NGOs funded by the Open Society Institute. The Open Society Institute established the international harm reduction program in 2000 to fund NGOs in 12 countries in the region. This effort reaches injecting drug users and commercial sex workers with information, education, counseling, referrals, and follow-up services. Integrating such programs into the national plan is problematic, in large part because of the stigma associated with injecting drug users and the perception that such programs support illegal activities.

Other groups also support harm reduction in the region, including the Red Cross (needle exchange), the Transnational AIDS/STD Prevention Among Migrant Prostitutes in Europe Project (TAM-PEP) (commercial sex worker outreach and networks), the International Organization on Migration (commercial sex workers and injecting drug users), and Médecins Sans Frontières (clinical and harm reduction services). USAID supports demand reduction through school-based and other education programs for young people on the relationship between injecting drug use and HIV/AIDS.

Commercial sex workers are a high-risk group for HIV because of their multiple sexual partners and because of their exposure to concomitant sexually transmitted infections that facilitate HIV spread. Studies from India, Thailand, Western Africa, Uganda, and elsewhere have shown the cost-effectiveness of condom promotion, peer education, and availability of treatment for sexually transmitted infections for commercial sex workers (Global HIV Prevention Working Group 2002).

A related issue for many commercial sex workers in Eastern Europe and Central Asia relates to trafficking in women and girls, a phenomenon associated with the financial and social disruptions following the dissolution of the Soviet Union and with postconflict situations, including lack of governance, in parts of the region. In 1997 the International Organization on Migration estimated that such trafficking involved 175,000 women and girls from Central and Eastern Europe and the NIS, representing one-quarter of all women involved in such trade worldwide (IOM 2002). Experience in other regions of the world reveals the high vulnerability of trafficked women and children to HIV/AIDS and sexually transmitted infections. Little evidence for effective interventions and awareness is seen in Eastern Europe and

Central Asia. Most interventions are by NGOs, and integration of these programs into national HIV/AIDS activities is lacking. Stigmatization, marginalization, and legal barriers (prostitution is illegal throughout the region, and returning sex workers are often ostracized by home country authorities) complicate effective interventions.

The World Bank's comparative advantage in harm reduction includes its capacity to integrate different approaches into policy discussions in multiple sectors, including ministries of justice. Efforts could include providing nonlending (analytical and advisory) services and support for operational research in grant-, credit- or loan-supported projects to assess efficacy and cost-effectiveness of harm reduction and other prevention programs; involving NGOs working on harm reduction in policy dialogue at the country level; and, where allowed by governments, financing drug dependency treatment and rehabilitation programs, needle and syringe exchange programs, and outreach work with commercial sex workers and injecting drug users to reduce risk behavior among them. Most important, the World Bank needs to engage governments and local institutions in policy dialogue to recognize the public goods involved in providing special attention to injecting drug users and commercial sex workers and their partners, the bridges to the general population. Where legal reform has been applied during low-level epidemics (as it has in Switzerland), the spread of HIV spread has not been explosive. Where there has already been an explosion, harm reduction has helped reverse a growing epidemic (in New York City), albeit at high cost. Decriminalizing injecting drug users, commercial sex workers, and homosexuals should at least be considered. This legal reform-based approach has had success in Western European programs that address HIV/AIDS in highly marginalized populations (Open Society Institute and International Harm Reduction Development 2003).

Health Promotion and Education

Health promotion and education are widely recognized as necessary primary prevention approaches to HIV/AIDS as part of modern public health practice. These approaches in Eastern Europe are based primarily in the school system. Broader-based educational activities addressing out-of-school youth, the general public, health professionals, and policymakers are also needed.

Health Education for Young People

Education about HIV/AIDS is an important tool for informing young people about behaviors that put them at risk for HIV infection. Worldwide young people account for more than half of new HIV infections, with more than 2.5 million people between the ages of 15 and 24 diagnosed every year (UNAIDS 2002d). Young people are often ill informed about HIV/AIDS and vastly underestimate their risk of becoming infected. It is preferable that young people obtain information about potential prevention of HIV before becoming sexually active. Evidence from Uganda, where HIV incidence has declined measurably, suggests the effectiveness of education and increased availability of prevention tools to alter risky sexual behavior (USAID 2002).

Interventions with young people have been shown to be cost-effective in Western HIV prevention programs (Pinkerton, Cecil, and Holtgrave 1998). These strategies include:

- Peer programs, the effectiveness of which has been shown in industrial countries for developing safer sex norms among young men who have sex with men.

- Social marketing of condom use, safer sex, and other healthy behaviors.

- School-based sex education (lacking in most countries in Eastern Europe and Central Asia).

- Special services that attract young people to health services, peer counseling, and other services.

In Eastern Europe and Central Asia as well as in other regions, prevention interventions have been implemented through the school systems. Young people in most countries are required to attend school through early adolescence. In many countries prevention programs targeting students have been highly effective in reducing risk behavior that places them at risk for HIV (Global HIV Prevention Working Group 2002). All programs provide education and information about HIV transmission and prevention; some may also seek to change risk behaviors (promoting condom use and encouraging fewer sexual partners or the delaying of sexual intercourse until marriage).

Several surveys have found that awareness and knowledge of HIV/AIDS by young people in Eastern Europe is low (Amirkhanian, Tiunov, and Kelly 2001; Lunin and others 1995; Westhoff and others 1996). Although the evidence demonstrating the importance of early HIV prevention education is clear, many young people in the region remain at risk because they leave school early and may not be exposed to HIV–related information that may be delivered during their school careers.

Information on high-risk behaviors is also needed. Young people in Eastern Europe are becoming sexually active at an earlier age, and an increase in drug use has been observed (UNAIDS 2002d). Sexually active adolescents who use contraception to prevent pregnancy may also be reducing their risk of HIV if condom use is part of their contraceptive behavior. Contraception is often not used in parts of Eastern Europe, however, because of cost and lack of availability (Novotny, Haazen, and Adeyi 2003). Methods of facilitating access to condoms for young people (increasing access to health clinics that are receptive to young people, providing condoms at schools and youth clubs) need to be explored.

Providing focused skills training—teaching young people how to resist negative media and social influence, for example—is another important aspect of education (UNAIDS 1997b). Peer education has also been shown to be effective in reducing HIV risk behavior (Jemmott, Jemmott, and Fong 1998). Most programs for young people also include information about the risk of HIV transmission associated with injection drug use and how to prevent drug-related transmission. The importance of these programs lies in their ability to help develop positive intentions regarding sexual behavior before an adolescent's initiation into sexual activity. It is much easier to adopt preventive behaviors from the start than to try to change established behaviors. School-based programs can combine provision of information with social norms for positive behavior (Peersman and Levy 1998).

In a Rapid Assessment and Response Survey of young people in Eastern Europe conducted by UNICEF (2002a), about half of sexually active respondents reported using condoms. Some respondents reported that condom use is not necessary with "clean" partners; condom use was used primarily for contraception rather than for prevention of sexually transmitted infections. The survey found that HIV/AIDS, drug, and sex education was either nonexistent or inadequate from any source (schools, parents). It also found that young people would get tested for HIV if testing were free, anonymous, and accessible. Anonymous testing was usually not available in the respondents' communities. Many Eastern European and Central Asian countries are constrained in facilities and funding. But low-resource countries such as Uganda have produced interventions that have reduced the incidence of HIV (UNAIDS 2002c).

The evidence argues for inclusion of HIV/AIDS education in schools, but implementation of educational programs is often hampered by shortages of funds and a lack of trained teachers with current information (Torabi and others 2000), legal barriers, or social taboos. When conducted properly, however, school-based HIV/AIDS education has been found to be effective. A video-based educational intervention in Russian schools was successful in improving both knowledge scores and attitudes in school children (Torabi and others 2000). Educational programs have been successfully implemented in other regions with few economic resources, including Sub-Saharan Africa. These types of programs thus seem feasible for Eastern Europe and Central Asia. Education of young people or the general public must be accompanied by infrastructure changes that permit young people-friendly services, widespread availability of condoms at low prices, and social marketing of prevention-oriented behavior (that is, the use of mass media, including commercials, public service announcements, and billboards, to provide information).

The Bank's comparative advantage in the field of public informa-tion and health education is significant. Operational research to evaluate the penetration of such messages may be financed by Bank-supported programs. Cooperation across education, health, and social protection sectors is essential to reaching young people and other vulnerable groups with prevention messages, both as part of school education and as part of community-based education. Work-ing with educational teams, human development health profession-als within the World Bank need to identify best practices from other regions for possible adaptation to Eastern European and Central Asian countries. The Bank's greatest challenge may be in promoting collaborative work between ministries. Input into such cross-sec-toral programming could occur within national HIV/AIDS over-sight groups.

Education of the General Public

The epidemic in the region is concentrated among certain risk groups. Some of these groups are nearly invisible due to stigmatiza-tion. Others—sex partners of commercial sex workers, injecting drug users, and men who have sex with men—may not even recog-nize that they are at risk. Thus it is important for the general popu-lation to be informed about HIV/AIDS, partly to improve basic knowledge about real risks and partly to reduce the stigma associ-ated with risk for or infection with HIV. The general public should be informed about modes of transmission, prevention, and treat-ment options.

Social marketing is a proactive approach to noncommercial, pub-lic education on health issues designed to match public needs with products and services (Rogers 1983). It involves informational cam-paigns to diffuse socially beneficial ideas (such as condom use) that address the increases in the incidence of sexually transmitted dis-ease. Such campaigns have recently been used in Albania, Kosovo, and Romania. This may be a useful approach to the epidemic of sex-ually transmitted diseases in other parts of the region as well. In addition, it will be important to address the public's level of comfort with and trust of the health care system and the government in dealing with sensitive personal issues such as HIV and sexually transmitted diseases.

Social marketing of safer sex to the general public has been shown to be cost-effective in preventing HIV infection (Walker 2003). It should therefore be included in education programs in the region. In addition, access to condoms needs to be increased and their price lowered. Educational messages for the general public need strengthening, and practices among clinical providers who have first contact with patients at risk need improving. Given the high levels of literacy, expanding access to electronic media, and potential channels for transmission (television, radio, Internet) in Eastern Europe and Central Asia, the media may be a particularly important avenue for increasing the low level of knowledge about HIV/AIDS in the region.

Studies have already shown the efficacy of social marketing in the region. A survey conducted in Estonia, Georgia, Hungary, Poland, and the Russian Federation revealed that 72 percent of respondents learned about HIV/AIDS primarily through the media (Goodwin and others 2003). In Moscow, a social marketing campaign involved leaflets, television commercials, and advertisements in newspapers and magazines (UNAIDS 1997a). Eighty percent of 1,228 people surveyed reported having seen the campaign, 83 percent found the information important for someone their age, and 93 percent said they would support the introduction of sex education in schools.

The media can also propagate false information—reporting, for example, that a cure for AIDS exists. Messages about HIV/AIDS thus need to be monitored for accuracy and validity (Goodwin and others 2003; Dilley, Woods, and McFarland 1997). In addition, in some Eastern European and Central Asian countries, such as Poland, religious institutions (particularly the Catholic Church) may exert a strong influence on the media, which they use to oppose dissemination of the message that safer sex can help prevent HIV prevention (Danziger 1996).

Governments must play a role in educating the general public about HIV/AIDS through a clear political commitment. In the United States the HIV/AIDS epidemic was peaking in the late

1980s. At that time, most of the general public was not well informed about HIV/AIDS, and misconceptions were very common. The U.S. Department of Health and Human Services issued pamphlets to every household in the country providing frank information regarding the risks of transmission of HIV/AIDS and addressing some common misperceptions and myths about the disease and the epidemic (U.S. Surgeon General 1988).

Political commitment has been a key component in Thailand and Uganda, where national programs were implemented with national leadership and local support. This political leadership, often manifested through media approaches, is key to successful prevention interventions.

The Bank's comparative advantage in this area lies in its capacity to conduct policy dialogue with senior decisionmakers at the country level and in providing loans or grants for communications campaigns on HIV/AIDS. The Bank funds numerous communications activities, primarily related to health system reform. These activities are often used to explain the need for reform and citizens' rights and responsibilities under reform. They can also be used to provide specific information on HIV/AIDS. Information also needs to be specifically tailored to policymakers, risk groups, young people, and ethnic groups.

Employment Group Approaches

HIV/AIDS is a multisectoral crisis, necessitating intervention beyond the health sector. Prevention activities targeting health professionals, teachers, military personnel, and transport workers can be effective.

Health Care Providers

Health behavior, attitudes, and practices among the general public may be influenced by health professionals. Health care providers are often the first point of contact for at-risk or recently infected people. They must be able to marshal up-to-date information and provide caring treatment to people living with HIV/AIDS.

Health providers need training in HIV/AIDS care in order to:

- Ensure that they can recognize behavior that places people at risk for transmitting or contracting HIV.

- Demonstrate sensitivity in dealing with people with HIV/AIDS.

- Refer people with or at risk for HIV to appropriate specialty and social service resources.

- Treat people with HIV/AIDS with scientifically based (peer-reviewed) methodologies and drug regimens in order to minimize drug resistance.

- Prevent hospital-acquired infection from contaminated blood, reused needles, and unnecessary injection treatments.

To perform these activities, health care workers must be adequately informed about and sensitive to issues regarding HIV/AIDS, especially issues affecting members of marginalized risk groups. Data are needed on attitudes of health professionals toward HIV and risk group categories. Health professionals' attitudes contribute to stigmatization; interventions against stigmatization must include the health profession.

Universal precautions—wearing gloves and goggles, properly disposing of needles and syringes, and carefully handling blood and blood products—are necessary in all health care settings to prevent accidental transmission of HIV to health care workers or patients through reuse of needles, lack of sterilization procedures, or inappropriate disposal of medical waste.

The Bank's comparative advantage here is in support of training and retraining of health professionals, a common component of health system operations in Eastern Europe and Central Asia. This training could focus on:

- Reducing the stigma associated with HIV/AIDS and risk profiles.

- Updating practices for identifying, testing, treating, and referring people with sexually transmitted infections and HIV/AIDS, especially people with opportunistic infections.

- Recognizing the social needs of people with HIV/AIDS and developing referral mechanisms for them.

- Working with NGOs and advocacy groups to provide extended services and to lobby for appropriate expansion of health services for people with HIV/AIDS.

- Using HAART appropriately.

- Using injection therapies appropriately and properly disposing of medical waste, including needles and syringes.

Military Personnel and International Peacekeepers

People serving in the armed forces or in peacekeeping units are at above-average risk of contracting HIV. This group also serves as a bridge for introducing the virus into the general population (UNAIDS/WHO 2002). The risk of military personnel being infected by a sexually transmitted infection (including HIV) is estimated at two to five times that of civilians (UNAIDS 1998). The risk is particularly high for men serving in areas of high HIV prevalence. Forty-five percent of Dutch naval and marine personnel serving as peacekeepers in Cambodia reported having sex with commercial sex workers or other local people (UNAIDS 1998).

Little is known about the rates of infection among peacekeepers. The United Nations does not require mandatory testing of deployed soldiers, and countries vary in their policies on testing military personnel. A WHO study reported that 27 of 52 countries surveyed (representing 44 percent of the world's population) performed mandatory HIV tests as part of military recruitment. The situation in Eastern Europe and Central Asia is not known, but several countries in the region provide peacekeepers to the United Nations (D'Amelio and others 2001).

Some countries have implemented HIV education programs as a part of basic military training. These programs typically provide voluntary counseling and testing services, condoms, and HIV education and awareness training.

The United Nations recently passed Resolution 1308, which states that the increased risk of HIV infection for peacekeepers could jeopardize the purpose and success of their missions (Bazergan and Easterbrook 2003). Services provided to U.N. troops have been criticized for not taking cultural differences into account, and there is little evidence that specific interventions aimed at reducing HIV risk behavior among U.N. forces have succeeded. Nevertheless, given the evidence from successful behavior change interventions conducted among other high-risk groups, well-designed and -implemented interventions—including social marketing of condoms, treatment of sexually transmitted infections, and risk education—could be an important aspect of prevention programs for military and peacekeeping personnel, even in countries where the overall prevalence rate may be low. Future interventions with military personnel and peacekeepers should include baseline surveys of knowledge, attitudes, and behavior in order to track the epidemic in these groups and compare these measures with sentinel biological measures of HIV infection.

The Bank's comparative advantage here is in policy dialogue that encourages interministerial cooperation. Defense ministries need to be included in national HIV/AIDS coalitions or steering groups. The risks associated with peacekeepers need to be measured and understood as a potential entry point for HIV infection.

Truckers and Mariners

In the Baltics, Southeastern Europe, and elsewhere, high-risk behavior takes place along major transportation routes, including ports (World Bank 2003c; Novotny, Haazen, and Adeyi 2003). Increased rates of sexually transmitted diseases, including HIV and hepatitis B and C, have been documented in these settings. These corridors and ports are often the location for concentrated commercial sex work and injecting drug use. A study in Uganda found that 35 percent of truck drivers were HIV–positive (Nzyuko and others 1997). In South Africa 66 percent of truck drivers had had a sexually transmitted disease in the previous six months and 29 percent reported having had sex with commercial sex workers without a condom (Ramjee and Gouws 2002).

Eastern Europe and Central Asia's transportation corridors and port cities expose the region to these risks. Bulgaria, Croatia, Estonia, Latvia, Lithuania, and Poland may be particularly vulnerable, because of their proximity to main transportation routes to countries in which the rate of HIV infection has increased (Belarus, the Russian Federation, and Ukraine) or because they have busy international ports. Prevalence data on HIV infection among truck drivers in Eastern Europe and Central Asia are not available, but there are indications that some truck drivers and mariners engage in behavior that places them at risk for HIV infection.

An intervention to reduce risk behavior among truckers was implemented in Tanzania (Laukamm-Josten and others 2000). The intervention used peer education and condom promotion to reduce risk among truck drivers and their sexual partners. The intervention increased condom use by men from 56 percent to 74 percent; condom use by their female sexual partners rose from 51 percent to 91 percent. Similar results occurred in India, where an intervention provided truckers with condoms and targeted education about HIV ("sex without condoms is like driving without brakes") (Singhal and Rogers 2003).

The Bank's comparative advantage here lies in its capacity to conduct policy dialogue to increase the visibility of the sector as a risk group and to work with industry and civil society groups to improve services, provide risk reduction education, and promote risk reduction tools (such as social marketing of condoms in ports and along transport routes) that are best implemented outside of hospitals or standard clinical environments.

Health System Issues

The health system is the focus of several preventive opportunities. First, people already infected with HIV need counseling and referral. This referral may often involve HAART. For the most part, countries in Eastern Europe and Central Asia retain health systems that guarantee treatment for established illness. Providing HAART may represent a major economic burden. Nonetheless, strategies must be developed to respond to the increasing burden of people infected with HIV for whom HAART is indicated. Second, the treatment and prevention strategies necessary for sexually transmitted infections have a direct implication for prevention of HIV spread.

Providing Highly Active Anti-retroviral Treatment (HAART)

HAART has lowered mortality from AIDS in industrial countries. This therapy is available in many Eastern Europe and Central Asia countries, although it is not clear how widely available it is within each country or whether international standards for quality, monitoring effectiveness, and minimizing the emergence of drug-resistant forms of HIV are being followed.

HAART reduces the viral load of people infected with HIV and is associated with several potential prevention benefits. It may increase incentives for voluntary counseling and testing, reduce stigmatization, and reduce the risk of infection by lowering circulating viral loads and infectivity.

Several significant potential downsides are associated with making HAART more widely available, however. First, HAART may not reduce the incidence of HIV, because people who continue to live with infection and engage in risk behavior may fuel the epidemic. Second, the presence of a treatment that is (erroneously) perceived as a cure may make high-risk groups more prone to reduce prevention efforts. Third, inappropriate therapy, self-therapy, or counterfeit drugs used in HAART may lead to avoidable high rates of drug resistance, heavy burdens on health financing systems, and inappropriate therapeutic regimes resulting from financial deficiencies, all of which can reduce the benefits of HAART to the general population.

Preventing Sexually Transmitted Infections and Reducing the Risk of HIV

Information, education, and behavior change aimed at reducing sexually transmitted infections will also reduce the risk of HIV transmission. Ulcerative sexually transmitted infections may increase the risk of HIV transmission. Of concern is the fact that syphilis rates are rising in several Eastern European and Central Asian countries. The reported syphilis rate in the Russian Federation, for example, rose from 4.2 per 100,000 in 1987 to 277 per 100,000 in 1997 (Amirkhanian, Tiunov, and Kelly 2001).

Transmission of sexually transmitted infections in Eastern Europe and Central Asia is primarily heterosexual. The presence of gonorrhea or syphilis is an indicator of sexual behavior that places one at risk for HIV (Nicoll and Hamers 2002). Thus strategies developed to prevent and treat sexually transmitted infections can also target HIV/AIDS. Reporting of sexually transmitted diseases discovered among pregnant women and commercial sex workers is particularly important. These diagnoses provide an access point for HIV testing and related behaviorally based prevention. However, such testing programs and the surveillance systems in which reporting is required are generally weak and unsystematic.

Considerable evidence appears to support the need to strengthen and build capacity for prevention and care of sexually transmitted infections. Other strategies for linking approaches to sexually transmitted infection and HIV include conducting routine HIV screening of patients at sexually transmitted infection clinics. This strategy has been demonstrated to be cost-effective even in low HIV prevalence settings (Bos and others 2002). A community-level trial in Tanzania that provided training to health center staff in the treatment and management of sexually transmitted infection, antibiotics to patients, and outreach to sexual contacts reported a 40 percent reduction in HIV incidence (Grosskurth and others 1995).

People most at risk for sexually transmitted infection (such as commercial sex workers and men who have sex with men) may fear stigmatization or prosecution. These fears could be addressed through social marketing of beneficial products and services provided through the health system, with an emphasis on confidentiality or anonymity.

The evidence shows that treatment of sexually transmitted infection is a cost-effective means of preventing HIV infection (Walker 2003). The Bank has a significant comparative advantage in financing—through grants, credits, or loans—large-scale operations that could include service delivery, surveillance, and access to treatment of good quality. Communications activities within operations supported by the Bank could promote socially beneficial ideas that address the growing epidemics of sexually transmitted infection as an intervention opportunity for primary HIV prevention.

Controlling Tuberculosis in People with HIV/AIDS

HIV prevention is a priority for tuberculosis control, since worldwide almost half of people with HIV eventually develop tuberculosis. Prevention of active tuberculosis infection and treatment is also a priority to prevent and reduce co-illness and death in people with HIV.

All tuberculosis prevention and treatment activities are applicable regardless of HIV serologic status. However, special measures to expand and intensify tuberculosis case finding and cure, as well as preventive tuberculosis therapy (treatment of sputum-negative but exposed people using single drug therapy for up to six months), are needed in settings where HIV infection is concentrated, such as among injecting drug users, inmates, commercial sex workers, and contacts of newly identified HIV–positive tuberculosis patients. The ProTest initiative (see annex A), including voluntary counseling and testing and either treatment or preventive therapy, is likely to be cost-effective (http://www.who.int/gtb/policyrd/TBHIV.htm#ProTEST).

Tuberculosis prevention in people with HIV/AIDS involves a six-month course of isoniazid preventive treatment, which reduces the risk of developing active tuberculosis as much as 40 percent. However, this effect is unlikely to last after treatment, especially in high tuberculosis exposure settings, such as prisons. Complicating the public health approach to tuberculosis is the fact that more prolonged isoniazid preventive treatment often results in lower compliance and possible drug resistance. Thus this secondary prevention approach to tuberculosis should be used only as an individual preventive measure rather than as a large-scale population intervention.

The tuberculosis treatment of choice for people with HIV/AIDS is one of three variants of directly observed therapy, short-course (DOTS) for six to eight months. These regimens are clinically proven to result in high cure rates and low tuberculosis recurrence among people infected with HIV. As for chronic and multidrug-resistant tuberculosis cases, second-line drugs are used in specialized settings; cure rates are lower and costs much higher (Maher, Floyd, and Raviglone 2002). Emerging evidence suggests that community-based therapy for multidrug-resistant tuberculosis can reach high cure rates in poorer developing country settings (Mitnick and others 2003). Any attempt to provide treatment and care to multidrug-resistant tuberculosis cases should avoid doing so at the expense of the basic population-based DOTS approach, however. Tuberculosis patients found to be HIV–positive also need referral and possible care for AIDS along with tuberculosis treatment.

Sterling, Lehmann, and Frieden (2003) sought to determine the impact of the WHO's DOTS strategy compared with that of DOTS-Plus on tuberculosis deaths, mainly in the developing world. They used a study design of decision analysis with Monte Carlo simulation of a Markov decision tree, with data from people with smear-positive pulmonary tuberculosis. The analyses modeled different levels of program effectiveness of DOTS and DOTS-Plus and high (10 percent) and intermediate (3 percent) shares of primary multidrug-resistant tuberculosis while accounting for exogenous reinfection. The main outcome measure was the cumulative number of tuberculosis deaths per 100,000 population over 10 years. The findings led to the conclusion that, under optimal implementation, fewer tuberculosis deaths would occur under DOTS-Plus than under DOTS. If, however, implementation of DOTS-Plus were associated with even minimal decreases in the effectiveness of treatment, substantially more patients would die than under DOTS. The policy implications are that countries should be encouraged to establish effective DOTS programs before venturing into DOTS-Plus, DOTS-Plus should not be implemented in a way that draws financial resources or managerial attention away from DOTS, and tuberculosis/HIV surveillance should be strengthened, including testing all tuberculosis patients for HIV.

Meeting Social Service Needs

Improvement is needed in nonmedical services for people who test positive for HIV. Some people may be hesitant to discover their HIV status, because they believe that they have no recourse should they end up testing positive (Vermund and Wilson 2002). Adequate social and psychological counseling services for people with HIV need to be in place as testing resources become more widely available. These services can take many forms. They can be provided in the context of community centers that provide referrals, medication, information on housing, and care for sick people. These services could be provided by general or specific medical clinics or through social service agencies. Assessments should be conducted to determine the best vehicle for various groups (several approaches may be necessary). It will also be necessary to create a workforce able to provide these services, which may entail special recruitment as well as money for specialized training.

The development of social services that meet the needs of people with HIV/AIDS should occur simultaneously with the development of prevention services, voluntary counseling and testing services, and surveillance activities. It is essential that services be in place so that people newly diagnosed with HIV have access to information, social services, and medical treatment for AIDS–related diagnoses and full-blown AIDS.

The Role of Nongovernmental Organizations

NGOs provide the backbone for many of the harm reduction and social service support activities for people at risk for or living with HIV/AIDS in parts of the region (Novotny, Haazen, and Adeyi 2003). The Open Society Institute funds NGOs throughout the region to conduct harm reduction and outreach programs among injecting drug users and inmates. Some countries, such as Croatia, have small government offices that support NGO activities as part of national strategies (Novotny, Haazen, and Adeyi, 2003). Throughout the region USAID supports NGOs through project-oriented activities focusing on reproductive health, school-based education, social marketing of condoms, and other proven interventions. In several countries, such as Bulgaria, NGOs such as Médicins Sans Frontières provide direct medical care to isolated populations through outreach clinics; voluntary counseling and testing is sometimes also offered in such settings. Mobile populations may need such clinics because of their lack of official status and subsequent lack of access to government-financed medical care in many countries. In Rijeka, Croatia, the local government, using some national government funding and NGO implementation, provides services to injecting drug users and other vulnerable populations outside of official health system physical facilities.

Scaling up the project-oriented approach will be the responsibility of governments. The challenge is to retain the independent nature of NGO–delivered services while integrating these activities with national or regional goals for reducing risk and providing services to vulnerable populations.

Political and Social Issues

Several legal, political, and social barriers impede implementation of proven preventive actions against HIV/AIDS and tuberculosis epidemics. These barriers may justify revision of legal codes restricting access to publicly financed medical care so that the public good can be better served through treatment of HIV and tuberculosis in noncovered patients. Insuring treatment of dangerous public health threats such as these will help prevent spread to the general population. They thus need to be addressed through special exceptions to financing restrictions. If they are not, such restrictions may exacerbate the associated epidemics, thereby creating additional economic burdens on health systems.

Mobile and Minority Populations

Migrant and other mobile populations are at increased risk for HIV. Factors that contribute to this increased risk are structural factors, including poverty, marginal knowledge of health information, and a discontinuation of cultural beliefs that may have been protective against HIV infection (for example, religious and cultural sanctions against sexual promiscuity, drug use, and community disruption). A history of internal and cross-national conflicts contributes to this risk (Axmann 1998), as well as negative attitudes toward the groups most affected. These populations often also lack psychosocial and government health financing resources and thus have low utilization of health services (Soskolne and Shtarkshall 2002). In some European countries, 70 percent of sex workers are migrants. Because migrant and mobile populations are frequently not included in surveillance activities, information about their behavior is limited, constraining the ability to tailor prevention activities for them (Salama and Dondero 2001).

Interventions aimed at migrant and ethnic minority populations should be tailored to the characteristics of the group targeted. The Swiss Migrants Project is an example of a successful government-sponsored intervention aimed at reducing the HIV risk behavior of migrants (Haour-Knipe, Gleury, and Dubois-Arber 1999). The program's success was attributed to the fact that the intervention was delivered by trained community members, increasing the receptivity of the target audience. Other successful interventions in migrant communities have also used peer education (Kocken and others 2001). In creating programs targeting migrants, however, it is important not to contribute to fears about migrant populations or to increase stigmatization of these groups by identifying them as "high risk."

Ethnic minority populations can be at increased risk for HIV because of economic and educational factors as well as lack of social protection services. In the United States, for example, African Americans represent more than 50 percent of new HIV infections, although they represent only 12 percent of the population (U.S. CDC 2000). Evidence from the United States and Canada suggests that interventions targeting these groups can reduce risk. A meta-analysis of HIV prevention interventions conducted among 7,010 heterosexual African Americans found that behavioral prevention interventions significantly increased the rates of protective behavior

(Darbes and others 2002). Successful interventions included education and information; risk sensitization (for example, altering the perception of risk for HIV infection); and skill building (for example, teaching negotiation skills about condom use, improving communication skills about safer sex). Cultural sensitivity was also shown to be an important aspect of the interventions. It is likely that such evidence will support targeted efforts among Roma and other ethnic minorities in Eastern Europe and Central Asia.

Eastern Europe and Central Asia is home to 5–10 million Roma, a minority population that has been isolated and oppressed for centuries. Given their isolation and lack of trust of medical systems, few data are available on their behavior. Drug use among Roma populations appears to be increasing, however, especially among disaffected and unemployed young people. HIV prevalence among Roma youth in Budapest has been estimated at 5–20 percent; about 10 percent of young Roma injecting drug users in the Czech Republic are believed to be HIV–positive (Grund, Ofner, and Verbraeck 2002).

Evidence on the health needs of Roma indicate high burdens of infectious diseases, poor communication between Roma and health workers, and low use of preventive care (Koupilova and others 2001). Evidence on effective interventions among the Roma is lacking. The admission process into the European Union may offer an opportunity to improve conditions for Roma in Eastern Europe and Central Asia. However, lack of advocacy and the absence of research into effective health interventions are barriers to improved support for this marginalized population.

Regarding intravenous drug use and commercial sex work, harm reduction programs among the Roma are even more difficult to implement than for the general population because of the traditional difficulties these programs have with police agencies. Needle exchange and education of commercial sex workers are difficult to implement under any circumstance, but the longstanding suspicion of Roma by the police complicate legalization of these approaches even further. Repressive drug legislation will likely have an even greater adverse effect on prevention efforts among the Roma. Most outreach activities for commercial sex workers and injecting drug users do not address Roma populations, and many of the standard educational approaches will be ineffective because of cultural taboos. Drug dependency treatment programs have attracted Roma in Slovakia, but it is not clear whether repressive new legislation will permit utilization of such services (Grund, Ofner, and Verbraeck 2002). Romani leaders emphasize the need for culturally appropriate, community-based approaches.

Stigmatization

In Eastern Europe and Central Asia, as in other parts of the world, a high level of stigma is associated with HIV/AIDS. Stigma was identified as one of the most pressing items on the agenda for the world community (Piot 2000).

A recent review of interventions to combat HIV/AIDS stigma categorized types of interventions as information-based approaches, skills building, counseling approaches, or contact with affected groups (Brown, Macintyre, and Trujillo 2003). Most of the studies were conducted in the United States, but some took place in Sub-Saharan Africa, Thailand, and the United Kingdom. The results varied in terms of success in reducing stigma. The most successful studies reported positive change for short periods of time. Most of the studies aimed at changing individual-level behavior and were based on individual theories of behavior and attitude change.

Parker and Aggleton (2003) argue that stigma may be successfully fought only at the social and community levels. They advocate for the implementation of community-based interventions aimed at broad societal change. They acknowledge that such change requires widespread community changes—in issues concerning power and inequality, for example. The need for community change demands broad structural interventions, but, as Brown, Macintyre, and Trujillo (2003) note, no such interventions have been implemented. However, there seems to be an underlying agreement on the need for such a broad-based approach to the human rights issues that underlie stigma. In fact, in the U.N. Declaration of Commitment on HIV/AIDS (2001), 189 member nations committed themselves to "enact, strengthen or enforce legal measures to eradicate HIV–related discrimination and to protect the human rights of people with HIV/AIDS."

Discrimination against men who have sex with men is widespread in the region, and homosexuality is still illegal in many countries. Men who have sex with men often find themselves deeply closeted, and they may have become fearful of further testing approaches due to the lack of anonymity associated with earlier compulsory screening efforts in the region (Kelly and Amirkhanian 2003). Personal privacy and confidentiality safeguards need to be built into any surveillance or voluntary counseling and testing systems. The evidence base from industrial countries suggests that such safeguards will increase the rate of voluntary counseling and testing among high-risk populations and that this will subsequently support behavior change that will reduce HIV transmission (U.S. CDC 2003b).

Value for Money: Cost-Effectiveness of Interventions to Control HIV/AIDS

Even with the increasing availability of international grants, credits, and loans, countries have finite organizational resources to commit to HIV/AIDS in the short term. Priorities thus have to be set. Even where there are declarations of intention to do everything immediately, choices must be made in light of operational, capacity, and resource constraints, at least in the short term. The only question is whether those choices are explicit or implicit. Implicit choices are more convenient from a political perspective, since they raise no questions about tradeoffs or relative emphasis. However, fighting an HIV/AIDS epidemic, particularly a concentrated epidemic at low prevalence rates, requires political recognition of the potential for a major increase in HIV cases and the acceptance of the most effective combinations of prevention efforts.

In making resource allocation decisions, policymakers consider a range of issues. Ideally, they would consider the likely impact on the epidemic, or the centrality of any proposed intervention to the course of the epidemic (Jha and others 2001). In relative terms, for example, interrupting interventions among high-risk core transmitters, such as injecting drug users, is arguably a more efficient use of resources than preventing mother-to-child transmission in a concentrated epidemic that is driven by transmission among intravenous drug users. The public policy choice is seldom of a binary nature, however; often, it is a matter of relative emphasis that arises after negotiations among interest groups. From the point of view of effective and efficient use of resources, it becomes crucial to ensure that those negotiated sets of priorities are informed by valid data from surveillance (where is the problem and what is its size?), the cost-effectiveness of interventions (how much value for money from different interventions aimed at achieving the same outcome?), and feasibility.

Optimization models can inform the resource allocation process by helping estimate the maximum number of infections at any given budget level. They involve identifying population subgroups for intervention, estimating the proportion of these subgroups that can be reached, estimating the total number of new infections expected in each of these subpopulations, defining the set of HIV prevention interventions to be considered, estimating the unit cost of each intervention, and estimating the expected effectiveness of each intervention (World Bank 2002e). Due to the weaknesses in surveillance systems in Eastern Europe and Central Asia and the paucity of cost data on HIV/AIDS programs, these exercises require considerable guesswork. However, they are necessary in order to generate discussions, make assumptions explicit, and draw attention to the need for better data.

The international evidence on cost-effectiveness is limited in scope and often of questionable quality (Creese and others 2002).) After reviewing the cost and cost-effectiveness evidence on HIV/AIDS prevention programs in low- and middle-income countries, Walker (2003) concluded that the methods applied and results obtained raised questions about reliability, validity, and transparency. First, not all of the studies reported the methods used to calculate the costs; some failed to provide the data needed to allow the results to be recalculated. Second, methods varied widely, rendering different studies, even within the same country and program setting, largely incomparable. Third, even with consistent and replicable measurement, most results were not comparable because of the lack of a common outcome measure. There is an urgent need for well-crafted studies of cost and cost-effectiveness that will help in planning and decisionmaking. This is an area in which the World Bank has a comparative advantage.

Summary

Several important conclusions emerge from the lessons of the first two decades of the HIV epidemic in Eastern Europe and Central Asia:

• Effective prevention is complex; there is no "magic bullet." No single prevention approach or program can work in every subpopulation. Simplistic prevention approaches, such as providing information alone, are likely to prove ineffective.

• Effective prevention takes time; behavior change does not occur overnight. Putting the components into place to address the factors affecting risk and vulnerability requires planning, time, effort, and resources. Moving prevention efforts from a small pilot project to a national scale also takes time—to build capacity, address the changes required, and allow the efforts to have an impact.

• Prevention efforts must begin early, while HIV prevalence is still low, if countries are to avoid major epidemics. Once HIV has reached significant levels in a subpopulation, prevention efforts need to play catch-up with the epidemic, and an opportunity to keep HIV prevalence at low levels will have been lost. Efforts initiated earlier will prove much more effective in the long run and significantly reduce the ultimate burden HIV/AIDS presents to a country.

• Prevention must take a long-term perspective. The HIV/AIDS epidemic will be a long-term challenge for health and social systems.

An effective vaccine is not yet on the horizon. Failing to undertake proven multisectoral/multilevel preventive efforts on HIV/AIDS and tuberculosis will result in increased economic, medical, and social burdens from these largely preventable diseases.

The concept of focused prevention remains at the center of efforts to address the HIV/AIDS and tuberculosis epidemics in Eastern Europe and Central Asia. This entails:

- Providing political leadership and commitment.

- Interrupting transmission early among subpopulations at higher risk.

- Initially focusing prevention resources on people at higher risk or vulnerability but steadily expanding prevention efforts outward to reach those at lower risk.

- Creating a supportive environment within the general population and the health profession to address vulnerable subpopulations and to reach particularly high-risk, marginalized populations.

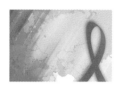

Overcoming Nonfinancial Constraints

Identifiable roadblocks, or constraints, impede successful implementation of programs to combat tuberculosis and HIV/AIDS. It is often suggested that these constraints are predominantly financial in nature—that is, that an increase in funding would remove the constraint. Often overlooked, however, is the question of how the money, once secured, would be applied to the problem and what issues would need to be addressed in the process (boxes D1 and D2). Put another way, if there were no constraints on financial resources, what nonfinancial constraints would limit the successful implementation of programs to control HIV/AIDS and tuberculosis? This question needs to encompass not only the internal institutions in a given country but also the external impediments created by a range of international development institutions, including the World Bank, the broader donor community, national governments, local populations, and specific sectors within countries.

Internal Constraints

Internal constraints exist at every level of government, as well as in the multiple layers of society. They include everything from political will to societal taboos and stigmas to inadequate technical capacity.

Box D1. Reaching Agreements in a Complex Setting: The Russian Federation's Tuberculosis and AIDS Control Project

By the end of 2002 the Russian Federation had more than 200,000 registered HIV cases, with the total number of infections estimated at 1 million. Without effective control, the epidemic would likely spread from the high-risk core transmitters to the bridge populations and the general population. The Russian Federation also had an epidemic of multidrug-resistant tuberculosis.

Despite the obvious need to act quickly, in early 2001 discussions over a large-scale project to control tuberculosis and HIV/AIDS reached an impasse. It took two years for the government and the World Bank to reach an agreement on countrywide implementation of effective tuberculosis and HIV/AIDS control strategies.

Why was the Russian Federation so slow to act in the face of these problems? How was the breakthrough accomplished? The shift was facilitated by the removal, through negotiations, of the following chokepoints in the decisionmaking process:

1. The leadership of the Russian health sector eventually became convinced that it was in the country's best interest to move forward: estimates and projections of the epidemic suggested potentially serious problems if the Russian Federation opted for business as usual through the traditional approaches to tuberculosis control and the patchy efforts to control HIV/AIDS (Ruehl, Pokrovsky, and Vinogradov 2002). Once senior Russian analysts became concerned about the potential demographic impact of the epidemic, decisionmakers began to view the epidemic as more than a problem affecting only socially marginalized groups.

2. In the mid-1990s international experts assumed that, faced with a fast-growing epidemic, the Russian Federation would automatically opt for the most effective interventions based on international guidelines. In fact, the Russian health establishment saw no need for major changes and preferred to develop its own protocols. The association of DOTS with less developed countries made it unacceptable to some parties. What turned out to be more feasible was an approach

Box D1. (continued)

designed specifically for the Russian Federation that represented a transition from the old system to a new one. The approach retained international guidelines at its core. This helped overcome institutional reluctance to change.

3. Some stakeholders in the Russian Federation had expressed opposition to the Bank's requirement that procurement by suppliers of therapeutic drugs be facilitated by the WHO's Green Light Committee. (The measure is essentially a quality assurance mechanism that helps ensure that countries meet technical criteria before they can have access to second-line drugs at preferential prices. It is intended to prevent the inappropriate use of second-line drugs, which could lead to resistance and the emergence of super drug–resistant strains of the tuberculosis bacillus.) The World Bank had taken extraordinary steps to enable the Russian Federation to procure quality-assured second-line drugs at low prices, but local drug suppliers perceived this as an attempt to stifle the Russian domestic market, creating a significant impasse. Ultimately, the World Bank reached an arrangement with the Russian government in which the government agreed to make the use of loan proceeds to purchase second-line tuberculosis drugs contingent on adherence to technical guidelines on quality, to be verified by the WHO. In addition, the Bank agreed that international competitive bidding could be used to create greater opportunities for Russian firms to compete. The Russian Federation would use its own funds to procure first-line drugs from the domestic market, with a buffer from the loan in case of budgetary shortfalls. This resolved one of the biggest obstacles to the agreement.

Source: Project Appraisal Document 21239-RU on a proposed loan to the Russian Federation for a tuberculosis and AIDS control project, March 10, 2003.

Box D2. Controlling Tuberculosis and HIV/AIDS in Moldova

After a decade of deteriorating economic performance, Moldova has shown the first signs of recovery, with rising GDP growth and a leveling off of poverty. Nevertheless, it remains the poorest country in Europe, with 55 percent of the population living on less than $2 per day.

The prevalence of HIV/AIDS in Moldova remained at a very low level during the first 10 years of the epidemic (less than 0.001 percent during 1987–96). Since the mid-1990s, however, there has been a surge in HIV infections, and HIV/AIDS prevalence has reached 0.2 percent among adults 15–49.

The tuberculosis epidemic has also increased over the past decade, due to worsening economic and social conditions that increase susceptibility to the disease, reduce access to care (including access to drugs), and lead to improper identification and treatment of people with tuberculosis. The incidence of tuberculosis increased 53 percent during the 1990s, and the trend has accelerated since then.

To address many of these issues, the government approved appropriate tuberculosis and HIV/AIDS strategies and designed the Moldova tuberculosis/AIDS program, with assistance from the Bank, the WHO, UNAIDS, UNICEF, the Dutch government, and the Swedish International Development Agency. It has sought funding to implement the program in the next five years. GFATM has already provided $5.2 million for fighting tuberculosis and AIDS. In June 2003 the Bank approved an International Development Association grant of $5.5 million for AIDS. USAID is expected to finance the tuberculosis program component with a grant of $4 million.

Working with vulnerable groups is a key component of Moldova's program, which includes identifying and then targeting interventions for injecting drug users, commercial sex workers, men who have sex with men, inmates, military personnel, and people who attend sexually transmitted infection clinics. The public health system lacks the capacity to carry out these outreach activities, while NGOs have experience working with these groups. It was therefore agreed that the Soros Foundation-

Box D2. (continued)

Moldova, which has been working for many years with NGOs that provide assistance to highly vulnerable groups, would manage these activities under the program. Ultimately, intensive collaboration between the government, NGOs, and international partners was an essential ingredient to the success of the process of establishing an appropriate program to control tuberculosis and HIV/AIDS in Moldova.

Source: Project Appraisal Document 25344-MD on proposed IDA grant to the Republic of Moldova for an AIDS control project, May 14, 2003.

Lack of Political Will and Recognition of the Problem

For years in Eastern Europe and Central Asia, denial of the problem by governments at all levels has been a significant constraint. Tuberculosis and HIV/AIDS were seen as problems of other parts of the world, and there was little empirical evidence to indicate they would become a problem in Eastern Europe and Central Asia. In a region going through the upheaval of transition from command to market economies, transferring resources to a potential problem was a difficult proposition. Governments, not without some logic, were able to make the case that in an environment of dwindling resources, dealing with tuberculosis and HIV/AIDS was not the most urgent priority.

The rise of tuberculosis and HIV/AIDS caught most of the region unprepared to address its impact on the health sector—and even less prepared to address its impact on the society at large. Like other regions before it, Eastern Europe and Central Asia has been slow to make the perceptual leap to begin to see HIV/AIDS and tuberculosis as more than "just" health problems. "Politicians, poli-

cymakers, community leaders, and academics have all denied what
was patently obvious—that the epidemic of HIV/AIDS would affect
not only the health of individuals, but also the welfare and well-
being of households, communities, and, in the end, entire societies"
(Barnett and Whiteside 2002, p. 5). Until there is a broader recognition of the magnitude of the potential crisis, countries will not be
willing to divert the necessary scarce resources.

Efforts have begun at changing the political and societal land-
scape. Increasingly, governments are acknowledging the importance
of HIV/AIDS and tuberculosis. Countries are developing national
programs for HIV/AIDS and tuberculosis control. International
financing is increasing, through grants, credits, and loans. Four
World Bank–financed projects on HIV/AIDS and tuberculosis are
at various stages of development in the region (in Belarus, Moldova,
the Russian Federation, and Ukraine). The Bank is also supporting
a range of analytical and advisory services in the region (see annexes
A, B, and E). Bilateral organizations (including the Canadian International Development Agency, the Department for International
Development, the Swedish International Development Agency, and
USAID); multilateral agencies (the eight cosponsors of UNAIDS);
and NGOs are supporting analytical and programmatic work on
HIV/AIDS and tuberculosis in the region. The discussions and
preparation processes leading up to these projects are themselves
vital in generating and building commitment among populations.
The projects generally rely on a broad battery of actions to address
political will, such as media campaigns that increase public awareness, multisectoral partnerships, training for workers and government staff, educational programs, and the development of new legal
frameworks. These actions help create broader recognition of the
threats posed by tuberculosis and HIV/AIDS and help build commitment to take action by the many players involved in implementing a program.

The political will that has helped bring about these projects
reflects progress in raising the level of awareness, but it is still only
the beginning of a long and challenging process. In Central Asia, for
example, although all five governments have either approved or are

considering approving strategic plans to combat HIV/AIDS, there is considerable room for improvement in the knowledge, attitudes, and practices of decisionmakers, opinionmakers, and health professionals to control the epidemic (Godinho, Lundberg, and Bravo 2002).

Success in transforming political will has been achieved through a process that includes:

- Demonstrating to senior analysts and policymakers the potential economic and epidemiological consequences of inaction.

- Obtaining the commitment of public funds, not just assurances of cooperation.

- Working closely with the health community, at the government, community, and rural levels, to raise awareness and prioritize issues.

- Building consensus through a multisectoral approach, with active involvement of ministries other than health ministries (education, justice, labor), as well as with NGOs, donors, and other partners.

- Building public awareness through public information campaigns, while recognizing that awareness alone is not sufficient.

Social Constraints and Stigmatization

One reason societies are slow to come to grips with the HIV/AIDS crisis is that many aspects of the problem are considered taboo or are frowned on by large segments of the population. It is difficult to raise awareness or build consensus on an issue that cannot be discussed openly. The problem is exacerbated by the fact that the majority of people affected by HIV/AIDS belong to groups that are marginalized by society.

The primary groups affected by HIV/AIDS—injecting drug users, commercial sex workers, and inmates—have limited access to community service infrastructures. They are also among the least likely to be well informed about safe sex practices and disease prevention. Since HIV/AIDS is still largely identified with these marginalized groups, there is a sizable element of society that is willing to adopt the logic of "it's not us, it's them." As long as the disease is perceived to affect only marginalized groups, it is not considered a threat to the larger community.

When HIV/AIDS does begin to expand beyond these groups, people are afraid to come forward—to be tested, to seek treatment, to take an activist position—because they fear being tarred as a member of one of these groups. Once the disease becomes stigmatized as something aberrant, people seeking treatment are discriminated against, and sources of support (funding, testing, and counseling) become scarce.

Personal and ethnic taboos create environments that are not conducive to treating these diseases. For example, the Roma, one of the poorest minorities in Europe (Ringold 2002), have historically avoided certain types of medical care, such as immunizations and Pap smears, for personal and cultural reasons (Acton and Mundy 1997). Involving such groups in dialogue on safe sexual practices is a complex and difficult process. Other religious and ethnic traditions can also affect willingness to participate in screening, prevention, and treatment.

Health care workers often carry the same biases and stereotypes regarding groups affected by the disease. Education and training for these front-line workers is a critically important first step.

Changing the environment of social constraints and stigmatization is fundamental to eliminating other constraints—to building political will and commitment, changing the legislative framework, and building capacity at the state and local levels. Critical steps that must be undertaken include:

- Achieving an understanding of social contexts and influences.

- Disseminating public information at every level. Campaigns on disease awareness, prevention, and treatment must be focused and strategically targeted to high-risk groups, including ethnic minorities and young people. In addition, efforts need to focus on destigmatizing the disease.

- Providing education, in schools and communities. Efforts need to include production of educational materials, such as brochures, booklets, and films.

- Conducting workshops and seminars for health workers, educators, and community groups.

Inadequate Capacity at the Community Level

Community infrastructure, or the lack thereof, is increasingly seen as having a major impact on health-related issues, including the implementation of tuberculosis and HIV/AIDS programs. Especially in countries with weak central governments, communities can play a vital role in education, treatment, and care. Unfortunately, many communities throughout the region are still recovering from the transition and lack the self-reliance required to support these initiatives. Efforts must be made to build capacity for community support and outreach programs.

Gender inequality is another critical factor that needs to be addressed. In many Eastern European and Central Asian countries, women remain excluded from decisionmaking bodies in community councils and local government. Low levels of education among women, particularly among some minorities, contribute to a low level of awareness about the disease, its transmission, and prevention (Paci 2002). At the same time, men are more affected than women in the current epidemiological profile; the epidemic has not become feminized.

High-risk behaviors such as unprotected sex, multiple partners, and injecting drug use have increased; the rigid social control of the past has eroded; and new common norms and values have yet to become firmly grounded (UNAIDS 2002d). Modifying risk behaviors in this context must become a multisectoral effort that involves schools, religious groups, and other community organizations. Community development and outreach programs should be built into project and components, and alliances with NGOs should be forged to foster community development.

Inadequate Institutional Capacity

Perhaps more than other constraints, institutional capacity varies dramatically across and within countries. Levels of poverty, education, technical development, ethnicity, geography, and myriad other factors all have critical importance in determining a society's ability to implement a program of prevention and treatment of tuberculosis and HIV/AIDS. That said, all countries in Eastern Europe and Central Asia must strive to improve their competence in certain key areas.

The World Bank has a wealth of experience in supporting and implementing complex projects, not only in health but in other social sectors and technical areas as well. To some extent, the problems associated with implementing any project reflect the level and sophistication of systems in place in a country. These include the ways in which people conduct business and the level of openness, corruption, and entrepreneurship in the society. Just as successful implementation of a project depends on these variables, creating or nurturing an environment for conducting a tuberculosis or HIV/AIDS control program depends on a confluence of associated factors.

These issues take on special importance when it comes to implementing effective intervention strategies (see annex C). For example, initiating and carrying out effective biological and behavioral surveillance systems depends on many factors, including the capacity to screen and analyze donated blood, conduct demographic and health surveys, maintain voluntary counseling and testing sites, and track and analyze mobile populations (Pisani 2002). Although some Eastern European and Central Asian countries have effective levels of these capacities, many others do not. Skilled scientists, laboratory technicians, demographers, analysts who can assess gaps in program management skills at the country level (gap analysis), educators, and counselors are all in short supply, as are the underlying infrastructures that support them. Also in short supply are the management skills necessary for planning and administering large and intersectoral programs at the national and local levels.

Harm reduction strategies require mechanisms and supplies that are often not available in Eastern Europe and Central Asia. Needle and syringe exchange projects require not only medical equipment but legal authorization and acceptance by the community. The same is true for drug dependency treatment programs and condom distribution among commercial sex workers. To gain acceptance and support, these issues need to be tackled at multiple levels—through government, education, and public awareness building.

Many parts of the region, including Bosnia and Herzegovina, Kosovo, and Tajikistan, also face postconflict issues that exacerbate the problems associated with HIV/AIDS. Not only have these conflicts drained resources and disrupted already deteriorating service infrastructures, they have generated new problems, including growing numbers of illegal migrants (who are unable or afraid to seek treatment), trafficked women and girls, and injecting drug users.

Another fundamental capacity issue is geographic, social, and financial access to services. In Tajikistan 80 percent of the country is mountainous, much of it remote. Providing health services in these areas is difficult. All of Central Asia is affected by this problem. In Slovakia 8–10 percent of the population are Roma (World Bank and others 2002), who live in sequestered settlements with limited access to healthcare. In Belarus injecting drug users are isolated and difficult to reach because of their infrequent contacts with the formal sector (World Bank 2002a). Physical access to testing and treatment is a critical first step that must be achieved throughout the region.

Underlying many of these problems are weaknesses in educational systems across the region. Education on HIV/AIDS is a critical component in the prevention of HIV/AIDS, through school prevention programs targeted at high-risk groups, awareness training, and dissemination of information to the public. Just as important, education is essential to train the community workers, counselors, and other health sector professionals required to address the crisis.

Other services are more dependent on financial resources. These include local and national distribution systems for pharmaceuticals, adequate laboratories, diagnostic infrastructures, and blood supply systems. The level of public information and communication provided also depends on financial resources.

Critical steps to raising institutional capacity include the following:

- Improving skills for gap analysis, program design, and management.

- Providing extensive education and training in testing and screening for tuberculosis and HIV infection; treatment and counseling; public education on tuberculosis and HIV/AIDS; program development and management; public information campaigns and disease awareness; and prevention programs that target commercial sex workers, injecting drug users, migrant workers, truckers, mariners, and peacekeepers.

- Developing distribution systems for pharmaceuticals and treatment, including in remote areas.

- Improving diagnostic infrastructures.

- Developing and disseminating public information materials.

Regulatory System Impediments and Other Legal Issues

Because of the nature of HIV/AIDS, the ways in which is transmitted, and the groups initially affected, an array of legal issues arises in implementing testing and treatment programs. For example, a key component in the harm reduction strategy is needle exchange, which is illegal in some countries. Many local regulatory frameworks do not allow key steps recommended under harm reduction practices. Legal issues also arise in prisons, a primary source of HIV transmission, where local regulations sometimes counter best practice for both tuberculosis and HIV/AIDS prevention and treatment.

Legal and regulatory frameworks are also critical in many peripheral areas of combating HIV/AIDS and tuberculosis. Often legal frameworks must be developed or altered to allow for the licensing and accreditation of health professionals and new educational programs. Insurance and risk pooling are other areas that need to be

updated and sometimes restructured to deal with the changes neces-
sitated by new treatments and expensive long-term regimens. A
range of societal issues, such as privacy and worker rights, also needs
to be addressed.

The laws governing the national and international procurement
and local distribution of therapeutic drugs also require attention.
International pressures have mounted on pharmaceutical companies
to provide antiretroviral drugs to developing countries at a lower
cost. However, the WTO Agreement on Trade-Related Aspects of
Intellectual Property Rights obligates its member states to grant
pharmaceutical patents, which increases the difficulty of providing
low-cost drugs to the neediest populations.

The Bank and other development agencies can assist countries in
the region by providing technical assistance in designing legal
frameworks, specifically with regard to harm reduction practices,
insurance, pharmaceuticals, and privacy, and prison initiatives or
reforms allowing a variety of steps, such as harm reduction, treatment, and care.

External Constraints

Addressing the internal constraints of 28 countries, with their broad
ranges of poverty, differing demographics and country landscapes,
and other factors, is a challenging task. In addition, a variety of
important external constraints affects the success of the objectives
and the progress of regional country programs on tuberculosis and
HIV/AIDS.

During the past five years, increasing attention and financial
resources have been allocated to programs for tuberculosis and
HIV/AIDS. Along with the attention and resources has come a wave
of heightened interest, new partners, and new strategies—galva-
nized in part by the adoption of the Millennium Development
Goals. Millennium Development Goal six states that by 2015 the
spread of HIV/AIDS, malaria, and other diseases will have been
halted and their spread begun to be reversed. Institutions that have

adopted the Millennium Development Goals face internal pressures to pursue these goals, even in countries in which the problem may not be as acute as in others and in which achieving the goals may be difficult (Goldman and Wright 2003).

With the rapid influx of funding, staff, and new programs, there is a risk of misapplying scarce resources. Some risks arise from the desire to disburse funds very rapidly—even in the absence of local capacity to absorb and manage them effectively. These risks include waste, inefficiencies, and the inappropriate use of drugs, which could lead to drug resistance (Reynolds and others 2003).

An important new player in the donor field is a new financing mechanism, the Global Fund to Fight AIDS, Tuberculosis and Malaria (GFATM). Endowed with growing financial resources, GFATM coordinates with the World Bank and a variety of other partners in the region to help halt and reverse the spread of tuberculosis and HIV/AIDS. Partly due to its newness, GFATM is still in the process of working through its approaches to country-level operations, and there have been delays in implementation (Summers 2002).

There is a potential conflict between a rapidly changing—and still relatively unknown—disease profile and the slow-moving processes that are characteristic of large international institutions such as the World Bank. Programmatic decisions at the Bank are generated by lengthy processes, such as the development of a Country Assistance Strategy, which sets out the basis targets for analytical, advisory, and lending services for a period of years. To be of maximum benefit to client countries, it is essential that institutions be vigilant to changes in the operating environment and ensure that there is enough flexibility in programmatic decisions that they are not locked into a single course of action and thus miss important developments in the epidemics.

Time and other institutional pressures also affect policy decisions. Preparation of grants, credits, and loans may require policy decisions before the evidence is in. To some extent, this problem is inherent in large and complex institutions.

Several areas call for reform:

- Increased attention should be given to disease surveillance and to estimates and projections of the economic impact of HIV/AIDS and tuberculosis in World Bank instruments such as Country Assistance Strategy and analytical activities in support of Poverty Reduction Strategy Papers, regardless of the prospect of lending to a given country.

- More should be done to ensure that Bank-supported operations are derived from, and integrated into, country strategies and programs.

- Greater emphasis should be placed on interagency coordination and country leadership. The coordination of programming and strategy is essential for the World Bank and its many international, national, and local partners in the region. It is critical, however, not to lose sight of the fact that agencies must support country-driven strategies and not become the primary drivers of a country's health policy. Agencies must cooperate and strategize with the country's health sector at the earliest stage possible, to design and implement programs that play to their respective strengths. Cofinancing of projects, sharing of research and data, and complementary planning are essential if impact is to be maximized.

Bureaucratic procedures are common in large organizations with complex missions, but the procedures for lending operations at the Bank remain excessively complex. Three areas in particular warrant attention:

- *Trust funds.* Lengthy and time-consuming application procedures, as well as restrictions on the use of consultant trust funds, create a disincentive for using this mechanism. Donor trust funds, which provide cofinancing or other forms of project support, often face significant delays due to the numerous clearances demanded by either the donor or the Bank.

- *Reporting and documentation requirements.* During the past several years, work on tuberculosis and HIV/AIDS, like much of the work in the social sectors, has increasingly become a patchwork of interrelated activities. These activities include projects, large and small grants, and trust funds, with requirements for inputs and clearances from multiple institutional units. Each type of activity has multiple internal and external time-consuming reporting and clearance requirements, which are frequently excessive and likely redundant.

• *Procurement.* Cumbersome procurement procedures and the need to reconcile different donors' procedures slow down implementation.

Recently, the Bank has undertaken a program of modernizing and simplifying procedures to address some of these issues. The Operations Policy and Country Services Department (OPCS), the Legal Department, and the Environmentally and Socially Sustainable Development Network (ESSD) have embarked on a program aimed at simplifying processing requirements for HIV/AIDS projects. This is a promising initiative.

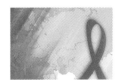

ANNEX E

Estimated Financial Resources Needed to Control HIV/AIDS and Tuberculosis in Eastern Europe and Central Asia

Scaling up HIV/AIDS and tuberculosis programs in Eastern Europe and Central Asia has resource implications. Estimating the costs of these programs can help policymakers obtain a more accurate picture of resource needs and plan accordingly. This is particularly important in countries in which public expenditures on health care are low and governments are under pressure to finance a growing basket of health services. This annex describes the resource needs for scaling up HIV/AIDS and tuberculosis programs, identifies potential resource gaps, and examines the implications for public expenditure and the role of donors.

Estimated Financial Resources Needed to Control and Treat HIV/AIDS

The materials presented in this section are from a joint World Bank–UNAIDS exercise that included consultations with country officials.

Methodology

The methodology for calculating HIV/AIDS resource needs is based on the resource needs model (Bollinger and others 2002).

This model, developed by the Futures Group, calculates the total national resources needed for HIV prevention, HIV/AIDS treatment, and orphan care programs.[11]

The model consists of three submodels: the prevention model, which includes the costs of 12 programs; the care and treatment model; and the orphan care model (tables E1 and E2).[12] The three main parameters of the model driving the calculations include unit cost estimates for each of the programs in the submodels, population or target groups, and coverage or access targets. The model includes parameters for all three parameters that can be adjusted based on expert opinion by country specialists and country-specific data.[13]

Unit cost estimates for prevention, treatment, and orphan care were obtained from 125 published and unpublished studies, most from Latin America and Sub-Saharan Africa. If the "default" values are used, the lower values are used for low-income countries and the values in the upper end of the range are used for middle-income countries. The population or target group calculations are made in a different way for the prevention and care models. For each prevention activity, the model first estimates the population target group in need of prevention services that could potentially have access to those services given existing infrastructure. For facility-based services, such as treatment for sexually transmitted diseases and voluntary testing and counseling services, access is estimated as the median of four variables: the percentage of the population with access to tuberculosis treatment (DOTS); essential immunizations (diphtheria, tetanus, and pertussis); attended births; and prenatal care.

The population target groups for other interventions consist of the relevant population subgroup (the population target group for school-based programs, for example, is children enrolled in school). The population needing care in a particular year is assumed to be equal to the number of people with HIV/AIDS who are newly symptomatic during that year. This number is estimated as equal to the number of people who would be expected to die of AIDS two years hence in the absence of treatment. People needing ongoing treatment (HAART and prophylaxis for opportunistic infections) include those who are newly symptomatic and those who were

Table E1. Prevention Activities, Target Populations, Default Coverage Rates, and Unit Costs

CATEGORY	ACTIVITY	TARGET POPULATION	DEFAULT COVERAGE (VARIES BY SEVERITY OF EPIDEMIC OR LEVEL OF ECONOMIC DEVELOPMENT)	DEFAULT UNIT COSTS (AT 2000 PRICES; MAY VARY BY REGION)
In-school youth	Teacher training, peer education	Primary and secondary students	10–33 percent of primary teachers 2–12 percent of secondary teachers	$26–$84 per primary teacher trained $15–$50 per secondary teacher trained
Out-of-school youth	Peer education	Out-of-school youth ages 6–11 and 12–15	10–50 percent of out-of-school youth	$8 per out-of-school youth reached
Commercial sex workers and their clients	Male and female condoms	Commercial sex workers	60 percent of commercial sex workers reached 60–80 percent condom use by those reached 5 percent are female condoms	$15.83 per commercial sex worker reached $0.10 per male condom distributed $1.00 per female condom distributed
Public and commercial sector condoms	Condom promotion	Single and married men with casual partners	Condoms used in 20–60 percent of casual sex acts 10–30 percent of married couples with casual partners use condoms in marital sex 70–80 percent of condoms distributed by public and commercial sector	$0.15 per male condom distributed

(Table continues on the following page.)

139

Table E1. (continued)

CATEGORY	ACTIVITY	TARGET POPULATION	DEFAULT COVERAGE (VARIES BY SEVERITY OF EPIDEMIC OR LEVEL OF ECONOMIC DEVELOPMENT)	DEFAULT UNIT COSTS (AT 2000 PRICES; MAY VARY BY REGION)
Social marketing of condoms	Condom promotion	Single and married men with casual partners	10–20 percent of condoms distributed through social marketing; 10 percent of condoms are female condoms	$0.12–$0.25 per male condom distributed; $1.00 per female condom distributed
Sexually transmitted infections	Treatment of sexually transmitted infections	Men and women with symptomatic sexually transmitted infections with access to health system services	60–100 percent of symptomatic sexually transmitted infection cases with access to health facilities; 60–100 percent of pregnant women with syphilis attending prenatal clinics	$8.34–$9.26 per sexually transmitted infection case treated; $0.91 per woman screened for syphilis at prenatal clinics; $8.34–$9.26 per syphilis case treated at prenatal clinics
Voluntary counseling and testing	Testing and counseling	Those desiring to be tested	Estimated as twice the number of people infected with HIV with access to health facilities, tested every five years	$10.60 per person counseled and tested
Workplace prevention	Condom promotion; Treatment of sexually transmitted infections	Men employed in the formal sector with casual partners; Men and women employed in the formal sector with symptomatic sexually transmitted infections	3–50 percent for peer counseling; 70 percent of employees with symptomatic sexually transmitted infections treated; 10 percent of all condoms distributed through workplace programs	$3.36 per employee reached with peer education; $8.34–$9.26 per sexually transmitted infection case treated; $0.10 per male condom distributed

Blood safety	Screening blood for transfusions	Units of blood required for transfusion	100 percent of blood tested	$4.88–$15.00 per safe blood unit available
Prevention of mother-to-child transmission of HIV	Testing Short-course antiretroviral treatment, replacement feeding	Pregnant women attending prenatal clinics HIV-positive pregnant women attending prenatal clinics	10–50 percent of women attending prenatal clinics tested 90 percent of those found to be HIV-positive accept treatment 50 percent of those found to be HIV-positive use replacement feeding	$3.80 per woman screened $18.70 per woman receiving antiretroviral regimen (includes drugs and service strengthening) $50 per women receiving formula
Mass media	Mass media campaigns	Country	Two to six campaigns per country per year	$490,000 per campaign
Harm reduction	Harm reduction programs	Intravenous drug users	25–75 percent of intravenous drug users	$3.21–$12.50 per person reached
Men who have sex with men	Peer counseling	Men who have sex with men	60 percent of men who have sex with men reached by peer counseling 60–80 percent condom use among those reached	$15.83 per person reached $0.10 per male condom distributed

Source: Bollinger, L., S. Bertozzi, J. Gutierrez, and J. Stover. 2002. Resource Needs Model for Estimating the Resource Needs for HIV/AIDS. The Futures Group. Available at www.futuresgroup.com.

Table E2. Unit Costs of Different Types of Treatment and Care (2000 dollars)

CATEGORY	ACTIVITY	ANNUAL COST PER PERSON
Palliative care	Symptomatic care and support provided to people near death	$75[a]
Diagnostic HIV testing	Testing of symptomatic patients before provision of prophylaxis for prevention of opportunistic infections or HAART	$5
Treatment of opportunistic infections	Medications and medical care for common opportunistic infections associated with HIV	$300[a]
Prophylaxis of opportunistic infections	Isoniazid (to prevent reactivation of latent tuberculosis) and cotrimoxazole (to protect against the pathogens responsible for pneumonia and diarrhea)	$32
HAART	Treatment with three antiretroviral drugs	$350–$2,900, depending on country wealth
	Laboratory testing to enable monitoring of HAART treatment	$140

a Lifetime cost.
Source: Bollinger, L., S. Bertozzi, J. Gutierrez, and J. Stover. 2002. Resource Needs Model for Estimating the Resource Needs for HIV/AIDS. The Futures Group. Available at www.futuresgroup.com.

receiving treatment the previous year. Newly symptomatic people initiating opportunistic infection prophylaxis without HAART are assumed to live two years on average; a Poisson distribution is used to determine the probability of death in a given year.

Coverage targets for prevention programs are calculated on the basis of several different factors, such as the level of coverage needed for program effectiveness, HIV prevalence rates, and the level of economic development. In low-income countries, coverage is naturally expected to be less than in middle-income countries with good health infrastructure. Coverage targets for treatment are calculated on the basis of available studies. Coverage rates are assumed to be higher for less sophisticated services. For example, more people would have access to palliative care than to HAART or treatment for opportunistic infections.

Caveats about the model should be noted. First, the model estimates feasible coverage targets assuming an ambitious expansion of current coverage unfettered by current financial resource constraints but without significant development in infrastructure. That is, no additional expenditures are provided for infrastructure development, with two exceptions. Expenditures on in-school education interventions consist mainly of teacher training; as such they represent investment in human infrastructure. A cost is also built in for strengthening the infrastructure needed to deliver interventions to prevent mother-to-child transmission. Second, the issue of sources of funding is not addressed. Instead, activities covered by all sources of funding are included. Costs related to capital and recurrent costs for surveillance activities are not included.

Using default parameters and other country-specific information, estimates were made for 135 countries in preparation for the U.N. General Assembly Special Session on AIDS (Schwartlander, Stover and others 2001). These initial estimates provided the basis for fine-tuning based on expert opinion and country-specific data. To produce country-specific estimates, a joint UNAIDS–World Bank workshop was organized in Minsk, Belarus, in November 2002. Representatives from eight CIS countries (Armenia, Azerbaijan, Belarus, Kazakhstan, the Republic of Moldova, the Russian Federation, Tajikistan, and Uzbekistan) attended the workshop.

During the workshop the unit cost estimates were revised for each country on the basis of expert opinion. Selected countries in the Baltics and Southeastern Europe were also sent the resource needs model for revising the unit cost data. Based on this information, country-level estimates were derived. The results presented here are mostly aggregates, with a few country-specific examples.

Results

Effective scaling up of essential programs for HIV/AIDS prevention, care, and treatment programs will require that funding from all source increase from about $300 million in 2001 to $1.5 billion by 2007 (see table E6). Needs by country will vary with the size of the population, the severity of the epidemic, and the unit costs of the prevention and care activities (see figure E1, which shows international assistance estimates, and table E1). Of the $1.5 billion required in 2007, three-fifths will be needed in the three countries with the largest populations (Kazakhstan, the Russian Federation, and Ukraine).

Distribution between Prevention and Care

In 2007, 40 percent of total funding will be needed for prevention; 55 percent for care and treatment; and 5 percent for policy, administration, research, and evaluation (figure E2). Provision of HAART, including laboratory monitoring costs, requires the largest percentage of funds (45 percent). Funding for HAART will need to increase from about $60 million in 2002 to more than $600 million by 2007. Three other important interventions together claim one-quarter of all funding requirements by 2007: treatment and prophylaxis for opportunistic infections (9 percent), workplace programs (7 percent), and condom promotion and distribution programs (6.3 percent).

The workshop in Minsk and the country review resulted in significant changes to the estimated resource requirements. The estimate of funding required for all interventions in 2007 rose 9 percent. Prevention needs were 38 percent higher and care needs 4 percent lower. Large increases were seen in the estimated costs of youth-focused programs (largely due to higher teacher training costs), management of sexually transmitted infections, and voluntary counseling and testing services. Estimated needs for workplace programs and mass media were significantly lower. The estimates of costs for laboratory monitory of HIV were somewhat lower in 2007.

Relative Emphasis on Selected Interventions

Despite the concentration of the epidemic among injecting drug users, fewer resources are allocated to programs for them than to programs targeting commercial sex workers and men who have sex with men. These estimates reflect not just the scale and unit costs

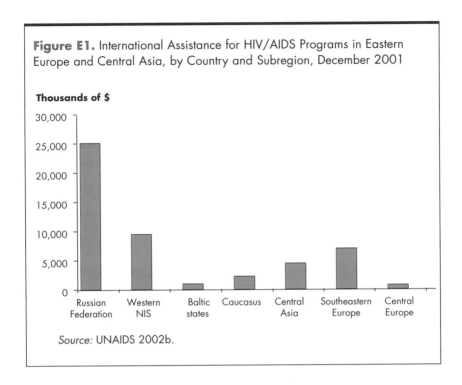

Figure E1. International Assistance for HIV/AIDS Programs in Eastern Europe and Central Asia, by Country and Subregion, December 2001

Source: UNAIDS 2002b.

but also what is considered feasible by country officials in terms of expanding the scale of their HIV/AIDS programs. The numbers reflect a certain degree of resignation by country participants. A more rapid expansion of harm reduction is not possible in some instances due to nonfinancial restraints, such as legal constraints. The problem cannot be tackled effectively without sufficient funding, but more funding cannot be used if the social and judicial constraints on harm reduction (for example) are not alleviated. Since many participants in the Minsk workshop are used to these constraints, they probably assumed that the constraints would remain, reducing their expectation of what could be done on some interventions by 2007. A key challenge is to alleviate nonfinancial constraints, such as judicial constraint on the expansion of harm reduction programs. This resource estimation exercise needs to be updated periodically to take account of changes in the operating environment and the scale of the epidemic.

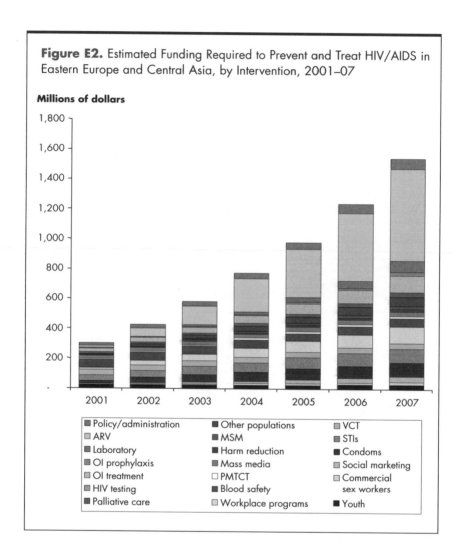

Figure E2. Estimated Funding Required to Prevent and Treat HIV/AIDS in Eastern Europe and Central Asia, by Intervention, 2001–07

Between 2001 and 2007 the resource needs for some prevention interventions (condom distribution, treatment of sexually transmitted diseases, interventions for commercial sex workers and their clients) increase rapidly, while the resource needs for others (interventions targeting young people) grow only marginally (see table E6). These differences are related largely to changes in coverage targets between 2001 and 2007. The resource needs model assumes that coverage increases over time. Increases in coverage are based on several assumptions, including current HIV prevalence rates and the economic classification of the country. Current HIV prevalence rates determine coverage rates, since in low-prevalence countries in order to effectively prevent new HIV infections only a certain percentage of the population needs to adopt a certain behavior. In addition, during the country consultations, coverage levels were refined after taking account of nonfinancial constraints for specific prevention interventions.

Future Costs of HAART

Country specialists made their best estimates of likely unit costs, coverage, and total expenditures for HAART in 2007. They expect Eastern European and Central Asian countries to spend more than $600 million on HAART, or 40 percent of the total HIV/AIDS budget. The country specialist estimates of annual unit costs varied from $200 to $3,600 per person, with an unweighted average of $1,600 per person. The specialists were asked to estimate prices and coverage for each year from 2001 through 2007. In general, they estimated that coverage would increase and unit prices, especially for pharmaceuticals, would decrease for low-income countries in Central Asia but increase or remain the same for most others, including Armenia, Kazakhstan, the Russian Federation, and Ukraine.

Making predictions as far into the future as 2007 requires considerable guesswork. The per person cost of HAART in Mexico declined about 90 percent between 1998 and 2002, due largely to the ability of the Mexican social security system to negotiate a lower price for drugs from pharmaceutical companies. In early 2002 a Thai pharmaceutical firm announced that it had succeeded in producing a single triple-therapy pill to be taken daily, which it expected to sell for $0.50 per dose ($185 a year). The TRIPS agreement remains a point of contention in international negotiations in the Doha Round on world trade. Pharmaceutical companies may have an interest in a high degree of price discrimination, often referred to as Ramsay pricing, maximizing their profits by selling at high prices in high-income countries and at lower prices in middle-

and low-income countries (Scherer and Watal 2002). These conditions make it difficult to predict future unit costs for this therapy. Moreover, if prices fall, coverage can be increased at the same total expenditure level.

Estimated Financial Resources Needed to Control and Treat Tuberculosis

Tuberculosis is likely to be the most common opportunistic infection and the number one killer of people with HIV/AIDS in Eastern Europe and Central Asia. The co-epidemic of HIV/AIDS and tuberculosis will add to the already growing problem of tuberculosis in the region. Since tuberculosis is spread through droplets released into the air by infected people, it is especially problematic among the poor and among institutionalized people, who typically live in crowded conditions.

Tuberculosis control is a public good with large externalities. It should be a priority for public funding in all countries in the region. In order to scale up tuberculosis programs it is useful to have information on potential resource needs.

Methodology

Resource needs for tuberculosis were calculated using the following methodology: First, for each country in the region, estimates were made for the increase in the number of tuberculosis cases between 2001 and 2007. Estimates were made for a low-case and a high-case scenario. The low-case scenario assumes that the incidence of tuberculosis without HIV will double between 1999 and 2010; the incidence of tuberculosis with HIV is assumed to be one out of three (33.3 percent). The high-case scenario assumes the same incidence rates, but the number of tuberculosis cases is larger because more people have HIV/AIDS.

Unit cost data on management of tuberculosis using current protocols were available only for the Russian Federation (WHO 2002a).

Costs there are high compared with other countries with similar income levels outside Eastern Europe and Central Asia. The higher costs reflect the longer average length of hospital stay for tuberculosis patients and mass screening, practices that are common in most other Eastern Europe and Central Asia countries as well. As countries in the region shift toward current WHO–approved methods for tuberculosis control, which call for less reliance on mass screening by x-ray and less hospitalization, these unit costs are likely to drop.

Unit costs from the Russian Federation were adjusted for each country in the region with gross national incomes of less than $1,000 in 2002 (Armenia, Azerbaijan, Georgia, Kyrgyz Republic, Moldova, Tajikistan, and Uzbekistan). Coverage was based on WHO targets for DOTS programs—that is, detection of 70 percent of new smear-positive cases and a cure rate of 85 percent. This methodology for calculating resource needs was used by the WHO's Stop Tuberculosis Department to calculate resource needs for 22 high-burden countries, including the Russian Federation, between 2001 and 2005 (Floyd and others 2002).

Results

Under the low-case scenario, resource needs increase from about $951 million in 2001 to $1.4 billion in 2007 (table E3). Under the high-case scenario, by 2007 annual tuberculosis control costs will be about $1.9 billion. These costs include the cost of treating all people detected with tuberculosis, including people with HIV.

Potential Resource Gaps and Policy Implications

By 2007 about $1.5 billion will be needed to treat HIV/AIDS and $1.9 billion to treat tuberculosis. These figures include some double counting, as the HIV/AIDS treatment costs include the costs of treating opportunistic infection treatment and prophylaxis.

These figures have implications for international assistance to countries in the region and for allocation of public resources for

Table E3. Estimated Cost of Treating Tuberculosis in Eastern Europe and Central Asia, by Country, 2001–07
(thousands of current dollars)

YEAR	LOW-CASE SCENARIO	HIGH-CASE SCENARIO
2001	951,262	951,262
2002	1,001,658	1,046,292
2003	1,056,837	1,151,150
2004	1,123,256	1,294,500
2005	1,198,338	1,464,213
2006	1,280,210	1,660,076
2007	1,368,337	1,883,076
Total	7,979,898	9,450,569

Source: World Bank estimates 2003.

health care within countries. The data do not easily allow disaggregation of current spending on HIV/AIDS. In particular, they do not allow disaggregation of HIV prevention, a public good, which should be financed from public resources. (Treatment of sexually transmitted infections that reduces HIV transmission is a private good with positive externalities.) Disease surveillance systems also yield important social benefits and can be considered public goods.

Most public funding for health care in Eastern European and Central Asia is still allocated to hospital care, followed by primary care. Although accurate estimates are not available, it is clear that public health spending has the least important place in government budgets.[14] Improving the allocative efficiency of public resources for health care, especially in the context of HIV/AIDS, is a critical issue that will need to be a high-priority item in the policy dialogue between the Bank and countries in the region. It would also be useful to collect better information on the source and flow of funds in countries in the region, perhaps through national health accounts (box E1).

The most recent comprehensive data on financing by cosponsors, bilateral agencies, and NGOs are for December 2001, when total international assistance for HIV/AIDS programs amounted to $51.7 million (UNAIDS 2002b) (table E4).

Table E4. International Assistance for National Responses to HIV/AIDS in Eastern Europe and Central Asia, by Program, December 2001

PROGRAM AREA	TOTAL INVESTED ($)	PERCENTAGE OF TOTAL
Prevention of HIV transmission related to intravenous drug use	14,668,169	28
Prevention among young people	12,277,935	24
Prevention among other vulnerable groups (men who have sex with men, sex workers)	8,136,884	16
Prevention of sexually transmitted diseases, HIV, mother-to-child transmission	7,239,456	14
Prevention through advocacy, information sharing, and networking	4,353,491	8
Care, counseling, and social support for people with HIV/AIDS	1,826,125	4
Blood safety	357,190	1
Surveillance, epidemiology, and research	106,000	0.20
Strategic planning, coordination, resource mobilization	1,475,239	3
Legal, policy, and ethical issues		
Condom programming	1,284,424	2
Total	51,724,913	100

Source: UNAIDS 2002b.

In 2002–03 GFATM became an additional source of funding on tuberculosis and HIV/AIDS in the region. Ten Eastern European and Central Asian countries received GFATM grants in rounds one and two of the proposal review process. Amounts granted for the first two years total $78.3 million, with $231.0 provided for the first five years (table E5).

The World Bank is also becoming an important source of funding for HIV/AIDS and tuberculosis control in Eastern Europe and Central Asia. Four World Bank–financed projects on HIV/AIDS and tuberculosis are at various stages of development in the region, in Belarus, Moldova, the Russian Federation, and Ukraine.

Box E1. Using National Health Accounts to Track the Source and Flow of Funds

National Health Accounts (NHAs) are a standard set of tables that present various aspects of a nation's health expenditures. They encompass total health spending in a country, including public, private, and donor expenditures. In addition to determining how much these financing sources allocate to health, NHAs carefully track the flow of funds from one health care actor to another, such as the distribution of funds from the Ministry of Health to each government health provider and health service. The NHA framework also allows for the analysis of data on targeted populations or disease-specific activities, such as expenditures related to maternal and child health or HIV/AIDS. This type of disaggregation of public and private spending by illness or disease category is critical, since HIV/AIDS and tuberculosis are infectious diseases for which private demand for treatment is likely to be lower than expected social benefits. This creates a rationale for public financing for prevention and treatment of infectious diseases.

Under the Latin America and Caribbean Regional initiative on HIV/AIDS (SIDALAC), data on public and private spending on HIV/AIDS were collected in 15 countries using the NHA framework. These data reveal that the region underspends on prevention and devotes too little attention to key groups (men who have sex with men, commercial sex workers, injecting drug users). Moreover, there is no clear pattern of spending priorities, and spending does not always match identified program priorities.

The Europe and Central Asia Region of the World Bank has recently launched an initiative in which several countries in the region will be developing NHAs. Given the importance of tuberculosis and HIV/AIDS in the region, these problems could be included in the NHA following the SIDALAC model.

Source: Abt Associates 2003; McGreevey 2003.

Table E5. GFATM Grants in Eastern Europe and Central Asia, 2002–2003
(millions of dollars)

COUNTRY	YEARS 1 AND 2	TOTAL (YEARS 1–5)
Armenia	3.2	7.2
Croatia	3.3	4.9
Estonia	3.9	10.2
Georgia	4.0	12.1
Kazakhstan	6.5	22.4
Kyrgyz Republic	5.6	18.3
Moldova (Round 1)	1.7	11.7
Romania	40.0	48.4
Ukraine (Round 1)	9.0	92.2
Serbia and Montenegro (Round 1, deferred funding)	1.1	3.6
Total	78.3	231.0

Note: Seven countries applied for but did not receive grants. Nine countries did not apply for grants.
Source: GFATM (www.theglobalfund.org) and Global Fund Observer.

In 2002 health care spending in Eastern Europe and Central Asia was $150 billion measured in purchasing power parity dollars (about $60 billion measured at 1997 exchange rates). A similar or larger amount is likely to be spent in 2007. Spending requirements for HIV/AIDS prevention and care, at $1.4 billion in 2007, would constitute no more than 1–3 percent of total health spending that year (depending on whether nominal exchange rate or purchasing power parity dollars are used). Detection and treatment of tuberculosis would consume 5–6 percent of health care costs. If efficiency were improved through adoption of cost-effective tuberculosis control strategies, these costs would likely drop significantly, to 2–3 percent of health expenditures.[15] These figures suggest that it should be feasible to finance the prospective level of spending required (although considerable donor support will be needed in the Caucasus and Central Asia). Much depends, however, on whether actions taken now can effectively restrain the epidemic, limiting the number of new infections. The high share of HAART spending in regional budget requirements, coupled with uncertainties about the cost of pharmaceuticals, leave a host of unanswered questions about financing.

Several countries in the region have effective social and private insurance arrangements that cover health care services. An ongoing policy debate may focus on the nature and extent of coverage these insurance institutions offer. Out-of-pocket spending may prove to be important in some countries as their health care financing systems evolve.

The most important source of finance is likely to be national and local governments, which will need to support the poor with subsidized health care and finance a large part of prevention services. Governments may prove to be the entities best able to negotiate for lower prices for HAART pharmaceuticals.

Aggregate figures mask huge disparities in per capita health expenditures across the region. During 1990–98 annual per capita spending on health care was $746 in Slovenia but just $13 in the Kyrgyz Republic and $6 in Tajikistan (World Bank 2002c). Some of the most economically challenged countries of the region (countries in the Caucasus, the Central Asian countries, and Moldova) are faced with a growing problem of HIV/AIDS. In these countries domestic and international resources will have to be mobilized for comprehensive HIV/AIDS prevention and treatment programs.

Summary

A substantial increase in resources is needed to fight HIV/AIDS in Eastern Europe and Central Asia. Funding needs to increase from about $300 million in 2001 to about $1.5 billion in 2007. That increase in resources requires that expenditures rise at a cumulative annual rate of 30 percent. This substantial rate of increase must be accompanied by staff training, testing equipment, better skills in policy and advocacy for behavioral changes, and a host of related practical responses. Increased funding can facilitate an effective response, but many organizational and operational changes must also take place to ensure effective implementation.

On a more optimistic note, fully scaling up the required program for HIV/AIDS care and support would require expenditures of no more than 3 percent of total likely health care spending in the region by 2007. This share suggests that resource mobilization is feasible.

Failure to mobilize resources and implement the care and support programs outlined here can only exacerbate the problems arising from the HIV/AIDS and tuberculosis epidemics. The likely future costs will be all the greater should there be delays in implementing these essential interventions.

Table E6. Estimated Resource Requirements for Preventing and Treating HIV/AIDS, by Activity, 2001–07 (thousands of dollars)

ACTIVITY	2001	2002	2003	2004	2005	2006	2007
Prevention-related activities	**231,454**	**296,514**	**357,374**	**419,018**	**483,124**	**548,869**	**619,705**
Youth-focused interventions	25,261	25,506	25,685	25,874	26,861	27,832	28,908
Interventions focused on commercial sex workers and their clients	1,648	3,848	6,444	9,496	12,949	16,890	21,373
Social marketing of condoms	3,691	7,200	11,691	16,422	21,791	27,366	34,572
Public and commercial sector condom provision	21,299	34,836	47,551	59,748	72,411	84,063	96,045
Improving management of sexually transmitted infections	35,924	45,048	54,450	64,058	73,816	83,680	93,618
Voluntary counseling and treatment	34,824	37,532	37,621	37,738	37,823	38,203	38,327
Workplace measures	14,906	31,747	45,797	59,801	73,789	89,082	106,783
Blood safety	54,422	54,469	54,587	54,642	54,701	54,765	54,833
Prevention of mother-to-child transmission	6,613	7,939	9,362	10,893	12,535	14,299	16,193
Mass media	19,646	21,443	23,319	25,195	26,972	28,669	30,445
Harm reduction programs	4,687	6,729	8,734	10,754	12,743	14,717	16,675
Interventions focused on men who have sex with men	2,382	4,829	7,466	10,303	13,334	16,551	19,935
Interventions focused on other vulnerable groups	6,150	15,388	24,669	34,093	43,397	52,752	61,996
Care and treatment services	**55,187**	**108,434**	**194,963**	**316,045**	**450,384**	**629,670**	**852,348**
Palliative care	11,855	13,705	15,801	18,322	21,222	24,570	28,305

Testing	43	79	133	213	323	467	642
Treatment of opportunistic infections	23,744	29,885	38,289	49,998	65,603	85,996	111,516
Prophylaxis of opportunistic infections	1,590	2,803	4,687	7,593	11,821	17,721	25,526
Lab HAART	1,057	3,655	8,559	16,810	29,665	48,419	74,270
Antiretroviral therapy	16,898	58,307	127,494	223,110	321,751	452,498	612,089
Policy, advocacy, administration, and research	**14,332**	**20,247**	**27,617**	**36,753**	**46,675**	**58,927**	**73,603**
Total	**295,548**	**418,037**	**570,557**	**760,002**	**965,873**	**1,220,994**	**1,527,212**

Source: Work performed by the UNAIDS Secretariat, the World Bank, and the Futures Group 2002.

157

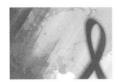

Notes

1.   Incidence refers to the number of new cases of HIV. Prevalence refers to the total number of cases of HIV.

2.   The eight cosponsors are the International Labor Organization (ILO); the WHO; the United Nations Development Programme (UNDP); the United Nations Children's Fund (UNICEF); the United Nations Educational, Scientific and Cultural Organization (UNESCO); the United Nations Office on Drugs and Crime (UNODC); the United Nations Population Fund (UNFPA); and the World Bank.

3.   The five elements of DOTS are political commitment to effective tuberculosis control; case detection among symptomatic patients self-reporting to health services, using sputum-smear microscopy; a standardized treatment regimen of six to eight months of short-course chemotherapy with first-line antituberculosis drugs, administered under proper case management conditions, including direct observation; uninterrupted supply of all essential antituberculosis drugs; and establishment and maintenance of a standardized recording and reporting system, allowing assessment of treatment results.

4.   The Gini coefficient is a number between zero and one that measures the degree of inequality in the distribution of income in a

given society. In a society in which everyone received exactly the same income, the Gini coefficient would be zero. In a society in which one person received 100 percent of income and the rest of the society earned nothing, the Gini coefficient would 1.0.

5. The low-case and high-case prevalences for the Russian Federation and Ukraine were slightly different because, by some unofficial estimates, both countries are already at or close to the 1 percent prevalence level. For these countries, the low case was taken as 1.5 percent and the high case was taken as 2 percent.

6. These costs are based on country consultations conducted to estimate the resource needs for HIV/AIDS prevention and treatment programs in Europe and Central Asia. For details on the workshop and the data, see annex E.

7. The total fertility rate refers to the average number of children a woman would bear over her lifetime if she experienced the current age cohort–adjusted fertility rates for specific years. The replacement level is a total fertility rate of 2.14. Life expectancy describes mortality levels in a given population at a particular point in time, as measured in years of life. It is affected by childhood and adult mortality rates. The lower the death rate, the more people survive throughout an entire age cohort and the greater the number of years they live.

8. According to the models developed by the Futures Group, as many as 60 percent of HIV/AIDS cases can be averted by implementing the package of prevention activities, provided a certain level of coverage is achieved.

9. Public health prevents epidemics and the spread of disease, protects against environmental hazards, prevents injuries, promotes and encourages healthy behaviors and mental health, responds to disasters and assists communities in recovery, and ensures the quality and accessibility of health services. Essential public health serv-

ices include monitoring health status to identify and solve community health problems; diagnosing and investigating health problems and health hazards in the community; informing, educating, and empowering people about health issues; mobilizing community partnerships and action to identify and solve health problems; developing policies and plans that support individual and community health efforts; enforcing laws and regulations that protect health and ensure safety; linking people to needed personal health services and ensuring the provision of health care when otherwise unavailable; ensuring a competent public health and personal health care workforce; evaluating effectiveness, accessibility, and quality of personal and population-based health services; and researching new insights and innovative solutions to health problems (U.S. CDC 1995).

10.   Sensitivity refers to how accurate a test is in detecting true positive cases among those tested. Specificity refers to how well a test correctly identifies people who are not infected (Dawson-Saunders and Trapp 1994).

11.   The Futures Group based the model on work done by Lilani Kumaranayake and Charlotte Watts, staff members of the London School of Hygiene and Tropical Medicine, and meta-analyses of cost-effectiveness studies managed by Bernhard Schwartlander, the former manager of strategic information at UNAIDS and the current director of HIV/AIDS programs at the WHO.

12.   The 12 programs in the prevention model include interventions with young people, interventions with sex workers and their clients, interventions with men who have sex with men, social marketing of condoms, public and commercial provision of condoms, improved management of sexually transmitted diseases, voluntary counseling and testing, workplace programs, blood safety programs, prevention of mother-to-child transmission, mass media campaigns, and harm reduction programs. The care and treatment model includes palliative care, treatment of opportunistic infections, diagnostic HIV testing, prophylaxis for opportunistic infection in symp-

tomatic patients, and HAART and its associated laboratory support. Orphan care includes care in orphanages, community assistance, and subsidies for school expenses.

13. In its initial 2001 formulation, the model added a flat 10 percent of prevention costs to cover administrative, research, monitoring, and evaluation costs. In the revised version used for Eastern Europe and Central Asia, the model adds 5 percent of total direct prevention, care, and treatment costs to cover these costs.

14. This information was derived from recently completed public expenditures reviews (PERs), social sector expenditure reviews, and health sector studies, specifically, the Romania Public and Institutional Expenditure Review (PIER) (2002), the Kyrgyz Republic PER (2003), the Georgia PER (2002), the Belarus Health Sector Note (2002), and the Ukraine PIER (2002).

15. Twenty countries in Latin America and the Caribbean spent a similar share of health expenditures on HIV/AIDS in 2000. They have HIV/AIDS prevalence levels similar to those in Eastern Europe and Central Asia.

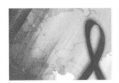

References

Abt Associates. 2003. "Understanding National Health Accounts: The Methodology and Implementation Process. Primer for Policymakers." PHRPLus Project. Abt Associates, Bethesda, Md.

Acton, M., and G. Mundy, eds. 1997. *Romani Culture and Gypsy Identity*. Hertfordshire: University of Hertfordshire Press.

Adeyi, O., R. Hecht, A. Soucat, and E. Njobvu. 2001. "AIDS, Poverty Reduction and Debt Relief." UNAIDS and World Bank. Geneva and Washington, D.C.

Ainsworth, M., L. Frasen, and M. Over. 1998. "Confronting AIDS: Evidence from the Developing World." World Bank Policy Research Report. Oxford University Press. New York.

Ainsworth, M., and W. Teokul. 2000. "Breaking the Silence: Setting Realistic Priorities for AIDS Control in Less Developed Countries." *Lancet* 356 (9231): 35–40.

Allen, S., A. Serufilira, J. Bogaerts, P. Van de Perre, F. Nsengumuremyi, C. Lindan, M. Carael, W. Wolf, T. Coates, and S. Hulley. 1992. "Confidential HIV Testing and Condom Promotion in Africa: Impact on HIV and Gonorrhea Rates." *Journal of the American Medical Association* 268 (23): 3338–3343.

Amirkhanian, Y.A., J.A. Kelly, A.A. Kukharsky, O.I. Borodkina, J.V. Granskaya, R.V. Dyatlov, T.L. McAuliffe, and A.P. Kozlob. 2001.

"Predictors of HIV Risk Behavior among Russian Men Who Have Sex with Men: An Emerging Epidemic." *AIDS* 15 (3): 407–412.

Amirkhanian, Y.A., D.V. Tiunov, and J.A. Kelly. 2001. "Risk Factors for HIV and Other Sexually Transmitted Diseases among Adolescents in St. Petersburg, Russia." *Family Planning Perspectives* 33 (3): 106–112.

Anderson, R.M. 1999. "Transmission Dynamics of Sexually Transmitted Infections." In K. Holmes, P. Sparling, S. Lemon, P. Piot, and J. Wasserheit, eds., *Sexually Transmitted Disease*. New York: McGraw-Hill.

Axmann, A. 1998. "Eastern Europe and Community of Independent States." *International Migration Quarterly Review* 36 (4): 587–607.

Barnett, T. 2003. "Economic and Social Impacts of the HIV/AIDS Epidemic in Eastern Europe and Central Asia." Draft paper prepared for the United Nations Development Programme, New York.

Barnett, T., and A. Whiteside. 2002. *AIDS in the Twenty-First Century: Disease and Globalization*. London: Palgrave Publications.

Bazergan, R., and P. Easterbrook. 2003. "HIV and UN Peacekeeping Operations." *AIDS* 17 (2): 278–279.

Bell, C., S. Devarajan, and H. Gersbach. 2003. "The Long-Run Economic Costs of AIDS: With an Application to South Africa." World Bank, Human Development Network, Washington, D.C.

Bloom, D., and J. Lyons. 1993. "Economic Implications of AIDS in Asia." United Nations Development Programme, Regional Bureau for the Asia and the Pacific, New Delhi.

Bloom, D.E., River Path Associates, and Sevilla Jaypee. 2002. "Health, Wealth, AIDS and Poverty." Paper prepared for the Asian Development Bank and UNAIDS.

Bollinger, L., S. Bertozzi, J.P. Gutierrez, and J. Stover. 2002. "Resource Needs Model for Estimating the Resource Needs for HIV/AIDS." Futures Group, Washington, D.C.

Bonnel, R. 2000. "Economic Analysis of HIV/AIDS." Unpublished document. World Bank, Africa Region, Washington, D.C.

Borgodoff, M., K. Floyd, and J. Broekmans. 2000. "Interventions to Reduce Tuberculosis Mortality and Transmission in Low- and Middle-Income Countries." *Bulletin of the World Health Organization* 80 (3): 217–227.

Bos, J.M., W.I. van der Meijden, W. Swart, and M.J. Postman. 2002. "Routine HIV Screening of Sexually Transmitted Disease Clinic Attenders Has Favourable Cost-Effectiveness Ratio in Low HIV Prevalence Settings." *AIDS* 16 (8): 1185–1187.

Brown, L., K. Macintryre, and L. Trujillo. 2003. "Interventions to Reduce HIV/AIDS Stigma: What Have We Learned?" *AIDS Education and Prevention* 15 (1): 46–69.

Brown, T., B. Franklin, J. McNeil, and S. Mills. 2001. *Effective Prevention Strategies in Low HIV Prevalence Settings.* Arlington, Va.: Family Health International.

Burrows, D. 2001. "A Best Practice Model of Harm Reduction in the Community and in Prisons in Russian Federation." Health, Nutrition, and Population Discussion Paper. World Bank, Washington, D.C.

Center for Strategic and International Studies. 2002. "Mobilization and Coordination." Washington, D.C.

Coates, T.J. 2000. "Efficacy of Voluntary HIV–1 Counseling and Testing in Individuals and Couples in Kenya, Tanzania, and Trinidad: A Randomised Trial." *Lancet* 356 (9224): 103–112.

Commission on Macroeconomics and Health. 2001. "Constraints to Scaling Up Health Interventions. Country Case Study: Chad." Working Paper WG5:18, HIV/AIDS. June. Geneva

Commonwealth of Independent States. 2002. "Urgent Response of Member States of the Commonwealth of Independent States to HIV/AIDS Epidemics." Approved by Council of the Heads of Government May 30.

Cox, H., and S. Hargreaves. 2003. "To Treat or Not to Treat? Implementation of DOTS in Central Asia." *Lancet* 361 (March 1): 714–715.

Creese, A., K. Floyd, A. Alban, and L. Guinness. 2002. "Cost-Effectiveness of HIV/AIDS Interventions in Africa: A Systematic Review of the Evidence. " *Lancet* 359 (May 11): 1635–1642.

Cruciani, M. 2001. "The Impact of Human Immunodeficiency Virus Type 1 on Infectiousness of Tuberculosis: A Meta-Analysis." *Clinical Infectious Diseases* 33 (11): 1922–1930.

D'Amelio, R., E. Tuerlings, O. Perito, R. Biselli, S. Natalicchio, and S. Kingma. 2001. "A Global Review of Legislation on HIV/AIDS: The Issue of HIV Testing." *Journal of Acquired Immune Deficiency Syndrome* 28 (2): 173–179.

Daniel, T. 1991. "Mycobacterial Diseases." In J. Wilson, E. Braunwald, K. Isselbacher, R. Petersdoff, J. Martin, A. Fauci, and R. Koot, eds. *Harrison's Principles of Internal Medicine*. 12th ed. New York: McGraw-Hill.

Danziger, R. 1996. "An Overview of HIV Prevention in Central and Eastern Europe." *AIDS Care* 8 (6): 701–707.

Darbes, L.A., N. Crepaz, C. Lyles, G.E. Kennedy, L. Zohrabyan, G. Peersman, and G.W. Rutherford. 2002. "Meta-Analysis of HIV Prevention Interventions in African-American Heterosexuals in the U.S." Paper presented at the Fourteenth International AIDS Conference, Barcelona, Spain, July 12.

Dawson-Saunders, B., and R.G. Trapp. 1994. *Basic and Clinical Biostatistics*. 2nd ed. Norwalk, Conn.: Appleton and Lange.

Defy, H. 2002. "Infrequent Injecting Drug Users: Research and Interventions with Young People at Risk of HIV, with Special Focus on CEE/CIS and the Baltics." Unpublished document. September. UNAIDS, Vienna.

Dehne, K.L., V. Pokrovsky, Y. Kobyshcha, and B. Schwartlander. 2000. "Update on the Epidemics of HIV and Other Sexually Transmitted

Infections in the Newly Independent States of the Former Soviet Union. " *AIDS* 14 (Suppl. 3): S75–S84.

Des Jarlais, D., M. Marmor, P. Friedmann, S. Titus, E. Avile, S. Deren, L. Torian, D. Glebatis, C. Murrill, E. Monterroso, and S.R. Friedman. 2000. "HIV Incidence among Injection Drug Users in New York City, 1992–1997: Evidence for a Declining Epidemic." *American Journal of Public Health* 90 (3): 352–359.

Des Jarlais, D., M. Marmor, D. Paone, S. Titus, Q. Shi, T. Perlis, B. Jose, and S.R. Friedman. 1996. "HIV Incidence among Injecting Drug Users in New York City Syringe-Exchange Programs." *Lancet* 348 (9033): 987–991.

Dilley, J.W., W.J. Woods, and W. McFarland. 1997. "Are Advances in Treatment Changing Views about High-Risk Sex?" *New England Journal of Medicine* 337 (7) (August 14): 501–502.

Domok, I. 2001. "Factors and Facts in Hungarian HIV/AIDS Epidemic, 1985–2000." *Acta Microbiologica et Immunologica Hungarica* 48 I (3–4): 299–311.

Dye, C., S. Scheele, P. Dolin, V. Pathania, and M.C. Raviglione. 1999. "Consensus Statement. Global Burden of Tuberculosis: Estimated Incidence, Prevalence, and Mortality by Country. WHO Global Surveillance and Monitoring Project." *Journal of the American Medical Association* 282 (7): 677–686.

Dye, C., B. Williams, M. Espinal, and M. Raviglione. 2002. "Erasing the World's Slow Stain: Strategies to Beat Multidrug-Resistant Tuberculosis." *Science* 295 (March 15): 2042–2046.

Einhorn, B. 1998. "The Impact of the Transition from Centrally Planned to Market-Based Economies on Women's Employment in East Central Europe." In E. Date-Bah, ed., *Promoting Gender Equality at Work*. London: Zed Books.

Espinal, M., S.J. Kim, P.G. Suarez, K.M. Kam, A.G. Khomenko, G.B. Migliori, J. Baez, A. Kochi, C. Dye, and M.C. Raviglione. 2000. "Standard Short-Course Chemotherapy for Drug-Resistant

Tuberculosis: Treatment Outcomes in Six Countries." *Journal of the American Medical Association* 283 (19): 2537–2545.

Espinal, M., K. Laserson, M. Camacho, Z. Fusheng, S.J. Kim, R.E. Tlali, I. Smith, P. Suarez, M.L. Antunes, A.G. George, N. Martin-Casabona, P. Simelane, K. Weyer, N. Binkin, and M.C. Raviglione. 2001a. "Determinants of Drug-Resistant Tuberculosis: Analysis of 11 Countries." *International Journal of Tuberculous Lung Diseases* 5 (10): 887–893.

Espinal, M., A. Laszlo, L. Simonsen, F. Boulahbal, S.J. Kim, A. Reniero, S. Hoffner, H.L. Rieder, N. Binkin, C. Dye, R. Williams, and M.C. Raviglione. 2001b. "Global Trends in Resistance to Antituberculosis Drugs." World Health Organization–International Union against Tuberculosis and Lung Disease Working Group on Anti-Tuberculosis Drug Resistance Surveillance. *New England Journal of Medicine* 344 (17): 1294-1303.

European Centre for the Epidemiological Monitoring of AIDS. 2002. "HIV/AIDS Surveillance in Europe. End-Year Report 2001." Report 66. Institut de Veille Sanitaire, Saint Maurice, France.

Field, M., and M. Twigg, eds. 2000. *Russia's Torn Safety Nets: Health and Social Welfare During the Transition.* New York: St. Martin's Press.

Floyd, K., L. Blanc, M. Raviglione, and J.W. Lee. 2002. "Resources Required for Global Tuberculosis Control." *Science* 295 (March 15): 2040–2041.

Frieden, T. 2002. "Can Tuberculosis Be Controlled?" *International Journal of Epidemiology* 31(5): 894–899.

Gayle, H.D. 2003. "Curbing the Global AIDS Epidemic." *New England Journal of Medicine* 348 (May 1): 1802–1805.

Global HIV Prevention Working Group. 2002. "Global Mobilization for HIV Prevention: A Blueprint for Action." http://www.gatesfoundation.org/connectedpostings/hivprevreport_final.pdf.

Godinho, J., E. Lundberg, and M. Bravo. 2002. "Concept Note for the Central Asia HIV/AIDS Study." Unpublished document. World Bank, Europe and Central Asia Region, Washington, D.C.

Goldman, P., and A. Wright. 2003. "Achieving the Human Development MDGs in Eastern Europe and Central Asia." Unpublished document. World Bank, Europe and Central Asia Region, Washington, D.C.

Goodwin, R., A. Kozlova, A. Kwiatkowska, L.A.N. Luu, G. Nizharadze, A. Realo, A. Kulvet, and A. Rammer. 2003. "Social Representations of HIV/AIDS in Central and Eastern Europe." *Social Science and Medicine* 56 (7): 1373–1384.

Grosskurth, H., F. Mosha, J. Todd, E. Mwijarubi, A. Klokkeand, and K. Senkoro. 1995. "Impact of Improved Treatment of Sexually Transmitted Diseases on HIV Infection in Rural Tanzania: Randomised Controlled Trial." *Lancet* 346 (8974): 530–536.

Grund, J.P. 2001. "A Candle Lit from Both Sides: The Epidemic of HIV Infection in Central and Eastern Europe." In Karen McElrath, ed., *HIV and AIDS: A Global Vi*ew. Westport, Conn.: Greenwood Press.

Grund, J.P., P.J. Ofner, and H.T. Verbraeck. 2002. "Drug Use and HIV Risks among the Roma in Central and Eastern Europe." Open Society Institute Working Paper. Budapest.

Hamers, F.F., and A.M. Downs. 2003. "HIV in Central and Eastern Europe." *Lancet* 361 (9362): 1035–1046.

Hamers, F.F., A. Infuso, J. Alix, and A.M. Downs. 2003. "Current Situation and Regional Perspective on HIV/IADS Surveillance in Europe." *Journal of Acquired Immune Deficiency Syndrome* 32 (Supplement 1): S39–S48.

Haour-Knipe, M., F. Gleury, and F. Dubois-Arber. 1999. "HIV/AIDS Prevention for Migrants and Ethnic Minorities: Three Phases of Evaluation." *Social Science and Medicine* 49 (10): 1357–1372.

Harvard Medical School and the Open Society Institute. 2001. "Review of Tuberculosis Control Program in Eastern Europe and the Former Soviet Union." Cambridge, Mass.

IOM (International Organization on Migration). 2002. "Migration Trends in Eastern Europe and Central Asia: 2001–2002 Review." New York.

Jack, W. 2001. "The Public Economics of Tuberculosis Control Health Policy." *Health Policy* 57 (2): 79–96.

Jemmott, J.B., L.S. Jemmott, and G.T. Fong. 1998. "Abstinence and Safer Sex HIV Risk-Reduction Interventions for African-American Adolescents: A Randomized Controlled Trial. " *Journal of the American Medical Association* 279 (19): 1529–1536.

Jha, P., N. Nagelkerke, E. Ngugi, J. Rao, B. Willbond, S. Moses, and F. Plummer. 2001. "Reducing HIV Transmission in Developing Countries." *Science* 292 (April 13): 224–225.

Kelly, J.A., and Y.A. Amirkhanian. 2003. "The Newest Epidemic: A Review of HIV/AIDS in Central and Eastern Europe." *International Journal of Sexually Transmitted Diseases and AIDS* 14 (6): 361–371.

Kocken, P., T. Voorham, J. Brandsman, and W. Swart. 2001. "Effects of Peer-Led AIDS Education Aimed at Turkish and Moroccan Male Immigrants in the Netherlands. A Randomised Controlled Evaluation Study." *European Journal of Public Health* 11 (2): 153–159.

Kongsin, S., and C. Watt. 2000. "Conducting a Household Survey on Economic Impact of Chronic HIV/AIDS Morbidity in Rural Thailand: Methodological Issues." AIDS and Economics Symposium, IAEN Symposium for Durban Conference on HIV/AIDS.

Koupilova I., H. Epstein, J. Holcik, and M. McKee. 2001. "Health Needs of the Roma Population in the Czech and Slovak Republics." *Social Science in Medicine* 53: 1191–1204.

Laukamm-Josten, U., B.K. Mwizarubi, A. Outwater, C.L. Mwaijonga, J.J. Valadez, D. Nyamwaya, R. Swai, T. Saidel, and N. Nyamuryekunge. 2000. "Preventing HIV Infection through Peer Education and Condom Promotion among Truck Drivers and Their Sexual Partners in Tanzania, 1990–1993." *AIDS Care* 12 (1): 27–40.

Lunin, I., T.L. Hall., J.S. Mandel, J. Kay, and N. Hearst. 1995. "Adolescent Sexuality in St. Petersburg, Russia." *AIDS* 9: S53–S60.

MacPherson, M.F, D.A. Hoover, and D.R. Snodgrass. 2000. "The Impact on Economic Growth in Africa of Rising Costs and Labor Productivity Losses Associated with HIV/AIDS." Harvard Institute for International Development, Boston.

Maher, D., K. Floyd, and M. Raviglione. 2002. "A Strategic Framework to Decrease the Burden of Tuberculosis/HIV." WHO/CDS/tuberculosis/2002.296.

McGreevey, W. 2003. "SIDALAC: Challenges and Opportunities." Futures Group, Washington, D.C.

McKee, M., J. Healy, and J. Falkingham, eds. 2002. *Health Care in Central Asia*. European Observatory on Health Care System Series. London: Open University Press.

Merson, M.H., J.M. Dayton, and K. O'Reilly. 2000. "Effectiveness of HIV Prevention Interventions in Developing Countries." *AIDS* 14 (Suppl. 2): S68–84.

Mitnick, C., J. Bayona, E. Palacios, S. Shin, J. Furin, F. Alcantara, E. Sanchez, M. Sarria, M. Becerra, M.C. Fawzi, S. Kapiga, D. Neuberg, J.H. Maguire, J.Y. Kim, and P. Farmer. 2003. "Community-Based Therapy for Multidrug-Resistant Tuberculosis in Lima, Peru." *New England Journal of Medicine* 348 (2): 119–2.

Nicoll, A., and F. Hamers. 2002. "Are Trends in HIV, Gonorrhoea and Syphilis Worsening in Western Europe?" *British Medical Journal* 324 (June 1): 1324–1327.

Novotny, T., D. Haazen, and O. Adeyi. 2003. "HIV/AIDS in Southeastern Europe: Case Studies from Bulgaria, Croatia, and Romania." World Bank Working Paper 4. Washington, D.C.

Nzyuko, S., P. Lurie, W. McFarland, W. Leyden, D. Nyamwaya, and J.S. Mandel. 1997. "Adolescent Sexual Behavior along the Trans-Africa Highway in Kenya." *AIDS* 11 (S1): 21–26.

Open Society Institute and International Harm Reduction Development. 2002. "Sex Worker Harm Reduction Iinitiative. Mid-Year Report. A

Guide to Contacts and Services in Central and Eastern Europe and the Former Soviet Union." Budapest.

Over, M., and P. Piot. 1993. "HIV Infection and Sexually Transmitted Diseases." In D. Jamison, W.H. Mosley, A.R. Measham, and J.L. Bobadilla, eds. *Disease Control Priorities in Developing Countries*. New York: Oxford University Press.

Paci, P. 2002. "Gender in Transition." World Bank, Europe and Central Asia Region, Washington, D.C.

Parker, R., and P. Aggleton. 2003. "HIV and AIDS–Related Stigma and Discrimination: A Conceptual Framework and Implications for Action." *Social Science and Medicine* 57 (1): 13–24.

Peersman, G., and J. Levy. 1998. "Focus and Effectiveness of HIV–Prevention Efforts for Young People." *AIDS* 12 (Suppl. A): S191–S196.

Phili, R., and E. Vardas. 2002. "Evaluation of a Rapid Human Immunodeficiency Virus Test at Two Community Clinics in Kwazulu-Natal." *South African Medical Journal* 92 (10): 818–821.

Pinkerton, S.D., H. Cecil, and D.R. Holtgrave. 1998. "HIV/STD Prevention Interventions for Adolescents: Cost-Effectiveness Considerations." *Journal of HIV/AIDS Prevention and Education for Adolescents and Children* 2: 5–31.

Piot, P. 2000. "Report by the Executive Director. Programme Coordinating Board." Joint United Nations Programme on AIDS, Rio de Janeiro, December 14–15.

Pisani, E. 2002. "Second-Generation Surveillance for HIV: The Next Decade." http://www.unaids.org/publications/documents/epidemiology/ surveillance/cdrom/surveillance guidelines/2nd generation surveillance/ 2nd gen eng.doc.

Pisani, E., G. Garnett, N. Grassly, T. Brown, J. Stover, C. Hankins, N. Walker, and P. Ghys. 2003. "Back to Basics in HIV Prevention: Focus on Exposure." *British Medical Journal* 326: 1384–1387.

Pitayanon S., S. Kongsin, and W.S. Janjareon. 1997. "The Economic Impact of HIV/AIDS Mortality on Households in Thailand." In David Bloom and Peter Godwin, eds., *The Economics of HIV and AIDS: The Case of South and South East Asia*. UNDP.

Powell, D. 2000. "The Problem of AIDS." In M.G. Field and J.L. Twigg, eds., *Russia's Torn Safety Nets: Health and Social Welfare During the Transition*. New York: St. Martin's Press.

Pozniak, A., R. Miller, and L. Ormerod. 1999. "The Treatment of Tuberculosis in HIV–Infected Persons." *AIDS* 13 (4): 435–445.

Ramjee, G., and E.E. Gouws. 2002. "Prevalence of HIV among Truck Drivers Visiting Sex Workers in KwaZulu-Natal, Africa." *Sexually Transmitted Diseases* 29 (1): L44–49.

Reichman, Lee B. 2002. *Timebomb: The Global Epidemic of Multidrug-Resistant Tuberculosis*. New York: McGraw-Hill.

Respess, R.A., M.A. Rayfield, and T.J. Dondero. 2001. "Laboratory Testing and Rapid HIV Assays: Applications for HIV Surveillance in Hard-to-Reach Populations." *AIDS* 15 (Suppl. 3): S49–S59.

Reynolds, S., T. Bartlett, T. Quinn, C. Beyrer, and R. Bollinger. 2003. "Antiretroviral Therapy Where Resources Are Limited." *New England Journal of Medicine* 348 (18): 1806–1809.

Rhodes, T., C. Lowndes, A. Judd, L. Mikahilova, A. Sarang, R. Rylkov, M. Tichonov, K. Lewis, N., Ulyanova, T. Alpatova, V. Karavashkin, M. Khutorksoy, M. Hickman, J. Parry, and A. Renton. 2002. "Explosive Spread and High Prevalence of HIV Infection among Injecting Drug Users in Togliatti City, Russia." *AIDS* 16: F25–F–31.

Rhodes, T., L. Mikhailova, A. Sarang, C. Lowndes, A. Rylkov, M. Khutorksy, and A. Renton. 2003. "Situational Factors Influencing Drug Injecting, Risk Reduction, and Syringe Exchange in Togliatti City, Russian Federation: A Qualitative Study of Micro Risk Environment." *Social Science and Medicine* 57: 39–53.

Rhodes, T., L. Platt, M. Davis, F. Filatova, and A. Sarang. 2002. *Behavioral Risk Factors in HIV Transmission in Eastern Europe and Central Asia: A Review*. Geneva: UNICEF/UNAIDS.

Rhodes, T., G.V. Stimson, N. Crofts, A. Ball, K. Dehne, and L. Khodakevich. 1999. "Drug Injecting, Rapid HIV Spread, and the 'Risk Environment': Implications for Assessment and Response." *AIDS* 13 (Suppl. A): S259–S269.

Ringold, D. 2000. "Roma and the Transition in Central and Eastern Europe." World Bank, Europe and Central Asia Region. Washington, D.C.

Robalino, D. 2002. "International Evidence on the Impacts of HIV/AIDS on Domestic Savings Rate." World Bank Policy Note. Washington, D.C.

Robalino, D., C. Jenkins, and K.E. Maroufi. 2002. "The Risks and Macroeconomic Impacts of HIV/AIDS in the Middle East and North Africa." Policy Research Paper 2874. World Bank, Middle East and North Africa Region, Human Development Group, Washington, D.C.

Roberts, M., B. Rau, and A. Emery. 1996. "Private Sector AIDS Policy: Businesses Managing AIDS: A Guide for Managers." AIDSCAP Project. Family Health International, Arlington Va.

Rogers E. M. 1983. *Diffusion of Innovations*. 3rd ed. New York: Free Press.

Rosenbrock, R., F. Dubois-Arber, M. Moers, P. Pinell, D. Shaeffer, and M. Setorn. 2000. "The Normalization of AIDS in Western European Countries." *Social Science and Medicine* 50: 1706–1629.

Rotily, M., C. Weilandt, S.M. Bird, K. Kall, H.J.A. Van Haastrecht, E. Iandolo, and S. Rousseau. 2001. "Surveillance of HIV Infection and Related Risk Behavior in European Prisons: A Multicenter Pilot Study." *European Journal of Public Health* 11 (3): 243–250.

Ruehl, C., V. Pokrovsky, and V. Vinogradov. 2002. "The Economic Consequences of HIV in Russia." World Bank, Moscow. www.world bank.org.ru.

Salama, P., and T.J. Dondero. 2001. "HIV Surveillance in Complex Emergencies." *AIDS* 15 (S3): S4–S12.

Scherer, F.M., and J. Watal. 2002. "Post–TRIPS Options for Access to Patented Medicines in Developing Countries." New Delhi: Indian Council for Research on International Economic Relations.

Schwartlander, B., P.D. Ghys, E. Pisani, S. Kiessling, S. Lazzari, M. Carael, and J.M. Kaldor, eds. 2001a. "HIV Surveillance in Hard-to-Reach Populations." *AIDS* 15 (Suppl. 3): S1–S3.

Schwartlander, B., J. Stover, N. Walker, L. Bollinger, J. Gutierrez, W. McGreevey, M. Opuni, S. Forsythe, L. Kumaranayake, C. Watts, and S. Bertozzi. 2001b. "Resource Needs for HIV/AIDS." *Science* 292 (20): 2434–2436.

Sharp, S. 2002. "Modeling the Macroeconomic Implications of a Generalized AIDS Epidemic in the Russian Federation." Ph.D. diss. University of Colorado, Boulder, Department of Economics.

Shell, R. 2000. "Halfway to the Holocaust: The Economic, Demographic and Social Implications of the AIDS Pandemic to the Year 2010 in the Southern Africa Region." Konrad Adenauer Stiftung Occasional Papers. Johannesburg, South Africa.

Shiffman, J., T. Beer, and Y.X. Wu. 2002. "The Emergence of Global Disease Control Priorities." *Health Policy and Planning* 17 (3): 225–234.

Singer, M. 1997. "Needle Exchanges and AIDS Prevention: Controversies, Policies, and Research." *Medical Anthropology* 18 (1): 1–12.

Singhal, A., and E.M. Rogers. 2003. *Combating AIDS: Communication Strategies in Action.* London: Sage Publications.

Smolskaya, T. 1999. "Injecting Drug Abuse in St. Petersburg." Paper presented at the national seminar AIDS and Mobility: New Policy Directions in Finland. University of Tampere, Tampere, Finland, June 11–12.

Somlai, A.M., J.A. Kelly, E. Benotsch, C. Gore-Felton, D. Ostrovski, T. McAuliffe, and A.P. Kozlov. 2002. "Characteristics and Predictors of

HIV Risk Behaviors among Injection Drug–Using Men and Women in St. Petersburg, Russia." *AIDS Education and Prevention* 14 (4): 295–305.

Soskolne, V., and R. Shtarkshall. 2002. "Migration and HIV Prevention Programmes: Linking Structural Factors, Culture, and Individual Behavior: An Israeli Experience." *Social Science and Medicine* 55 (8): 1297–1307.

Sterling, T.R., H.P. Lehmann, and T.R. Frieden. 2003. "Impact of DOTS Compared with DOTS-Plus on Multidrug-Resistant Tuberculosis and Tuberculosis Deaths: Decision Analysis." *British Medical Journal* 326 (March 15): 574–580.

Summers, T. 2002. *Challenges and Opportunities: A Report of the Committee on Resource Mobilization and Coordination.* Washington, D.C.: Center for Strategic and International Studies.

Tchoudomirova, K., M. Domeika, and P.A. Mardh. 1997. "Demographic Data on Prostitutes from Bulgaria: A Recruitment Country for International Migratory Prostitutes." *International Journal of Sexually Transmitted Disease and AIDS* 8 (3): 187–191.

Thomas, J.R. 2001. *HIV/AIDS Drugs, Patents, and the TRIPS Agreement: Issues and Options.* July. Report for the U.S. Congress. Congressional Research Service, Washington, D.C.

Torabi, M.R., J.W. Crowe, S. Shine, D.E. Daniels, and I. Jeng. 2000. "Evaluation of HIV/AIDS Education in Russia Using a Video Approach." *Journal of School Health* 70 (6): 229–233.

UNAIDS. 1997a. "Best Practice Summary Booklet: Safe Sex, My Choice." Russian Federation. Geneva.

———. 1997b. "Impact of HIV and Sexual Health Education on the Sexual Behavior of Young People: A Review Update." Report prepared for World AIDS Day. Geneva.

———. 1998. "AIDS and the Military." In UNAIDS, *Best Practice Collection.* Geneva.

———. 1999. *Best Practice Collection*. Geneva.

———. 2000. Economics in HIV/AIDS Planning: Getting Priorities Right. Geneva. Accessed on CD-ROM. UNAIDS/00.23E June.

———. 2002a. "Eastern Europe and Central Asia. National Responses to HIV/AIDS: Country Implementation Readiness Profile." January. Unpublished document. Geneva.

———. 2002b. "International Assistance for National Responses to the HIV/AIDS Epidemic in Eastern and Central Europe and Central Asia by 31 December 2001, as Reported by UNAIDS Cosponsors, Bilateral Agencies and NGOs." Geneva.

———. 2002c. "Knowledge Is Power: Voluntary HIV Counseling and Testing in Uganda."

———. 2002d. "Report on the Global HIV/AIDS Epidemic." Geneva.

———. 2002e. "Task Force Working Group Meeting on Substitution Treatment in Eastern Europe and Central Asia." Unpublished document. Vienna International Center, May 9–10.

———. 2003. "HIV/AIDS in the Eastern Europe and Central Asia Region: Economic and Social Impacts. Work in Progress." New York.

UNAIDS/WHO (World Health Organization). 2002. "AIDS Epidemic Update." December. Geneva.

UNDP (United Nations Development Programme). 2002. *Human Development Indicators*. New York.

———. 2003. "HIV/AIDS in the Europe and Central Asia Region: Economic and Social Impacts. Work in Progress." New York.

UNICEF (United Nations Children's Fund). 2002a. "Rapid Assessment and Response on HIV/AIDS among Especially Vulnerable Young People in South Eastern Europe." http://www.unicef.org/albania/finalrar.pdf.

————. 2002b. "Social Trends in Transition, HIV/AIDS and Young People, Quality of Learning in Schools." *Social Monitor* 21–33. Florence.

UNICEF/IOM (International Organization on Migration). 2002. "Overview of HIV/AIDS in South Eastern Europe. Epidemiological Data, Vulnerable Groups, Governmental and Nongovernmental Responses up to January 2002." Geneva.

USAID (U.S. Agency for International Development) and the Synergy Project. 2002. "What Happened in Uganda? Declining HIV Prevalence, Behavior Change, and the National Response. Project Lessons Learned Case Study." September. Washington, D.C.

U.S. CDC (Centers for Disease Control and Prevention). 1995. "Estimated Expenditures for Core Public Health Functions: Selected States, October 1992–September 1993." *Morbidity and Mortality Weekly Report* 44 (22): 421–429.

————. 2000. "HIV/AIDS Surveillance Report" *Morbidity and Mortality Weekly Report Surveillance Summaries* 12: 20–21.

————. 2003a. "Advancing HIV Prevention: New Strategies for a Changing Epidemic: United States, 2003." *Morbidity and Mortality Weekly Report* 52 (15): 329–332.

————. 2003b. "HIV Testing: United States, 2001." *Morbidity and Mortality Weekly Report* 52 (23): 540–545.

U.S. Surgeon General. 1988. "Understanding AIDS: America Responds to AIDS: A Message from the Surgeon General." Brochure prepared by the Office of the Surgeon General, Department of Health and Human Services, Washington, D.C.

Uuskula A., H. Silm, and T. Vessin. 2002. "Sexually Transmitted Diseases in Estonia: Past and Present." *International Journal of Sexually Transmitted Diseases and AIDS* 13: 184–191.

Valdiserri, R.O., R.S. Janssen, J.W. Buehler, and P.L. Fleming. 2000. "The Context of HIV/AIDS Surveillance." *Journal of Acquired Immune Deficiency Syndrome* 25 (S2): S97–S104.

Vannappagari, V., and R. Ryder. 2002. "Monitoring Sexual Behavior in the Russian Federation: The Russia Longitudinal Monitoring Survey 2001." April. Report submitted to the U.S. Agency for International Development. Carolina Population Center, University of North Carolina at Chapel Hill, North Carolina.

Vermund, S.H., and C.M. Wilson. 2002. "Barriers to HIV Testing: Where Next?" *Lancet* 360 (9341) (October 19): 1186–1187.

Vinokur, A., J. Godinho, C. Dye, and N. Nagelkerk. 2001. "The TB and HIV/AIDS Epidemics in the Russian Federation." World Bank Technical Paper 510. Washington, D.C.

Walker, D. 2003. "Cost and Cost-Effectiveness of HIV/AIDS Prevention Strategies in Developing Countries: Is There an Evidence Base?" *Health Policy and Planning* 18 (1): 4–17.

Westhoff, W.W., K. Klein, R.J. McDermott, P. Schmidt, and S.R. Holcomb. 1996. "Sexual Risk Taking by Moscovite Youth Attending School." *Journal of School Health* 66 (3): 102–105.

WHO (World Health Organization). 1997. "Guidelines for the Management of Drug-Resistant Tuberculosis." Geneva.

———. 2000a. "Anti-Tuberculosis Drug Resistance in the World." Geneva.

———. 2000b. "Guidelines for Establishing DOTS–Plus Pilot Projects for the Management of Multidrug-Resistant Tuberculosis." Geneva.

———. 2000c. "Strategy to Control Tuberculosis in the WHO European Region." WHO Regional Office for Europe. EUR/00/5017620. Geneva.

———. 2001. "An Analysis of Interaction between Tuberculosis and HIV/AIDS Programs in Sub-Saharan Africa." WHO/CDS/tuberculosis/2001.294.

———. 2002a. "Cost-Effective Tuberculosis Control in the Russian Federation. Results from the St. Petersburg Workshop." Geneva.

———. 2002b. "Developing a Strategic Framework for HIV–Related Tuberculosis in the WHO European Region." August 7 draft. Geneva.

———. 2002c. "DOTS–PLUS: Preliminary Results and Emerging Issues. Proceedings of the Meeting of the Stop Tuberculosis Working Group on DOTS–Plus for Multidrug-Resistant Tuberculosis." Tallinn, Estonia.

———. 2002d. "Global Tuberculosis Control: Surveillance, Planning, Financing." Geneva.

———. 2002e. "Guidelines for Applying to the Green Light Committee for Access to Second-Line Anti-Tuberculosis Drugs." WHO/CDS/tuberculosis/2001.286 Rev.1. Geneva.

———. 2002f. "Strategic Framework to Decrease the Burden of Tuberculosis/HIV." Geneva.

———. 2002g. DOTS Expansion Plan to Stop TB in the WHO European Region, 2002–2006. Copenhagen.

WHO/UNAIDS. 2000. "Guidelines for Second-Generation Surveillance." WHO/CDS/CSR/ECD/2000.5, UNAIDS/00.03E. Geneva.

WHO, UNICEF, UNAIDS, World Bank, UNESCO, and UNFPA (United Nations Population Fund). 2000. "Health: A Key to Prosperity. Success Stories in Developing Countries." http://www.who.int/inf–new/aids.htm.

World Bank. 2001. "HIV/AIDS in the Caribbean: Issues and Options." Latin America and the Caribbean Region, Washington, D.C.

———. 2002a. "Belarus Tuberculosis and AIDS Project." April. Project Appraisal Document. Europe and Central Asia Region, Washington, D.C.

———. 2002b. "Education and HIV/AIDS: A Window of Hope." Washington, D.C.

———. 2002c. "HNP Business Plan for Eastern Europe and Central Asia Region: Implementation of Health Projects 1990–2002." November. Unpublished document. Europe and Central Asia Region, Washington, D.C.

———. 2002d. "Moldova Tuberculosis/AIDS Project." Project Appraisal Document. Europe and Central Asia Region. Washington, D.C.

———. 2002e. "Optimizing the Allocation of Resources among HIV Prevention Interventions in Honduras." June. Latin America and the Caribbean Region, Washington, D.C.

———. 2002f. "Transition: The First Ten Years: Analysis and Lessons for Eastern Europe and the Former Soviet Union." International Bank for Reconstruction and Development, Washington, D.C.

———. 2002g. "Ukraine Tuberculosis and AIDS Control Project." Project Appraisal Document. Europe and Central Asia Region, Washington, D.C.

———. 2003a. "Health in Europe and Central Asia: Business Plan for 2003–2007." Unpublished draft document. Europe and Central Asia Region, Washington, D.C.

———. 2003b. "Russian Federation, Tuberculosis and AIDS Control Project." Project Appraisal Document. Europe and Central Asia Region, Washington, D.C.

———. 2003c. "Truck Drivers and Casual Sex: An Inquiry into the Potential Spread of HIV/AIDS in the Baltic Region." Europe and Central Asia Region, Washington, D.C.

———. 2003d. *World Development Indicators.* Washington, D.C.

———. Forthcoming. "Georgia: HIV/AIDS Policy Note." Europe and Central Asia Region, Washington, D.C.

World Bank, Open Society Institute, INEKO, and Foundation SPACE. 2002. "Poverty and Welfare of Roma in the Slovak Republic." April.

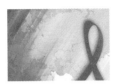

Index

183

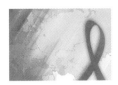

About the Authors

Olusoji Adeyi, MD, MPH, DrPH, is a lead health specialist in the Europe and Central Asia Region of the World Bank, where he serves as team leader for health programs in the Russian Federation and as regional focal point for HIV/AIDS Control. He has worked extensively on health system development in Central and Eastern Europe and in Africa. From 1999 to 2001 he served as senior advisor at UNAIDS in Geneva, on secondment from the World Bank, developing tools and strategies for linking HIV/AIDS control programs to poverty reduction strategies and debt relief as well as methods to improve the technical content of these programs. He is an adjunct assistant professor at the Johns Hopkins Bloomberg School of Public Health. He also serves as associate director of the AIDS Prevention Initiative in Nigeria, a program funded by the Bill & Melinda Gates Foundation through a grant to the Harvard School of Public Health.

Enis Baris, MD, MSc, PhD, is a senior public health specialist in the Europe and Central Asia Region of the World Bank, where he works as team leader for health projects in Azerbaijan, Bulgaria, and Turkey. He is also adjunct professor in the Department of Health Administration of the University of Montreal. At the World Bank he has worked extensively on health and development issues, including HIV/AIDS, in East Asia. Before joining the Bank he worked in Canada and for the WHO, where he conducted research on tobacco control, tuberculosis, and comparative analysis of health care systems in Eastern Europe, Latin America, and Sub-Saharan Africa.

Sarbani Chakraborty, MSc, PhD, is a health economist at the World Bank. She has worked on analytical and programmatic operations in several countries, including Georgia, the Kyrgyz Republic, and Slovakia. Her areas of technical expertise and interest include the public-private mix in the financing and delivery of health services, decentralization, provider payment systems, poverty reduction strategies, and the economic impacts of HIV/AIDS.

Thomas Novotny, MD, MPH, is the director of International Programs at the University of California, San Francisco, School of Medicine. He is a graduate of the University of Nebraska Medical Center, the University of California (San Francisco) Family Practice Residency Program, the U.S. Centers for Disease Control and Prevention's Preventive Medicine Residency Program, and the Johns Hopkins University School of Public Health. He has worked extensively as a World Bank public health consultant on health system reform, particularly in Eastern Europe. Dr. Novotny was a commissioned officer in the U.S. Public Health Service, serving as assistant surgeon general and deputy assistant secretary for International and Refugee Health. He has published widely on tobacco control, HIV/AIDS, and public health.

Ross Pavis, MFA, MPA, is an operations officer in the Europe and Central Asia Region of the World Bank. Heeee is a team leader of a social investment fund in Tajikistan and has worked on health projects in many countries in the region, including Albania, Croatia, Estonia, Romania, Slovenia, and Tajikistan. He has worked extensively with Roma, managing work programs in Hungary and Slovakia on capacity building, education, and poverty financed by the Institutional Development Fund and the Development Grant Facility.

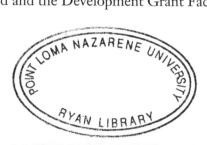